Ripping Up the Script

One couple's journey through infertility,
a man's perspective

Ripping Up the Script

One couple's journey through infertility,
a man's perspective

CHARLIE DRUCE

FOR MY DARLING, PARTNER THROUGH AND THROUGH

Introduction

It's Saturday morning. When our young son wakes up, around 7am, he hits the ground running. Sometimes that means jumping into bed with us, clambering over my head, stomach, groin, before he pouches down into the cosy slot between us. If we're lucky, we all get another half hour's snooze. Or a few moments' love-in when we perform an intense, wriggling kind of hug, usually reserved for a family of eels. But most often, it means jackknifing into action the plan he fixed up the previous evening and eventually fell asleep with, the one that is now mercilessly demanding our attention. Just like any other mum, dad, child combo up and down the land.

And for all this bonkers rushing around after our children, all these crazy collisions between work and home, we wouldn't have it any other way. Why? Because it's what we wanted. Wanted it for years. God knows it's not our right to have a child. But there's every good reason why parents or wannabe parents might think it is, and forgive themselves for thinking it too. Nothing else tastes quite like this.

It wasn't always like this, for my wife and me. Our son took his time to enter our lives, a nearly ten-year chunk of time. And during that time, we found ourselves having to play some challenging, unexpected roles – sometimes glued together more firmly, sometimes coming badly unstuck.

That's what this book is about: one couple's journey through infertility. The years of trying that got us to where we are now, told from a man's side of the fence (there's much written about infertility – books, blogs, articles, forum posts – but still, with notable exceptions, not much of it written by men).

Written, in part, for reasons to do with my own sense of that journey's closure. Only now, from the safety and sanity of several years' passing, can I look back and understand more about all that happened, and all that didn't. Yes, this all happened to me several years ago. It's been a while since I contemplated my lot in the small confines of a sample room, or watched – white-knuckled – as my wife ticked off her days with an IVF needle. Science, policy, treatments, drugs and public attitudes can all change (although surprisingly slowly, as each year passes). But the human experience of fertility, and its cruel counter-forces of infertility, remains the same – felt as deeply as anything we're capable of feeling.

But written also, I hope, because of what it may offer, just perhaps, for some of the many people who are starting, or have already begun, that difficult journey; their expectations around having a baby the natural way stretched to the very edges of what they can bear.

And there are a lot of us in the same leaky boat. An estimated one in seven UK couples experience difficulty in conceiving (sometimes you'll see this quoted as one in six), and in 2016, well over 50,000 women elected to have more than 68,000 cycles of IVF treatment between them. This was a 4% increase from 2015 to 2016.[1] Add to that figure the rising number of folks who choose to go overseas for their treatment, or who find another route to a child, adoption perhaps, or who manage their lives without – then that's a whole lot of people, couples and singles, touched by the wear and tear of this tough time in their lives.

I

Doing what comes naturally

When I stood up in front of our wedding guests, on one of those sunny with showers April afternoons, I felt, like most newlyweds, a strong and purposeful sense of the journey ahead. With my hand on my wife's shoulder, and the rest of the room beaming at us, I said that I could barely wait for the adventures of the present, let alone those of the future. And in amongst those adventures, of course, was the underlying bedrock of babies. Everyone in the room was warmly complicit, comfortable in their acceptance that here were two people, in love and together for the right reasons, perfectly free for now, but soon enough to be nicely weighed down with babies. The mapping out of children had already begun. A few weeks after the wedding, good friends of ours gave us two wedding presents. The first was tickets to a great evening out. The second was a dust buster. In their card they had written, 'This isn't for now, it's for the next stage.' The bottom drawer was already filling up. And so the dog-eared baby script was handed down to us, with us playing ourselves, the two leading roles. I was 33, my wife (she'll be called L from here on) exactly a year younger. The stage was set. Take out the marriage lines, and it's still, essentially, the same story. A couple team up for long enough and the expectation, usually, is the same. Babies, please.

L and I had met through the small world of our work in TV production. She was a Production Manager in a busy, often stressful commercials production company. I was co-running a smaller production company, not quite as stressful, but just as busy. As per the script, we worked hard, bought a new house and took some adventurous holidays. And after the usual while, L slipped out of the habit of birth control (the pill), something she had, like millions of other women around her, popped for most of her mature years (not least, in her case, for the ways it eased her period pains). We thought, quite naturally, that the pregnancy bit of our small-time drama would fall into place, that sooner or perhaps a little bit later, we would conceive and that L would fall pregnant. We were in control. Or at least we thought we were.

Nobody wants to ring any alarm bells in their lives unless it's urgent. And this didn't feel urgent. The fact that time was passing and that starting a family wasn't proving as easy as falling off logs didn't scare us. It's not like that, at least not to begin with. I see it now in others, when a friend or colleague tells me of the time it's taking them, and of the difficulty they're having. Just like we did, they're allowing that sense of self-protection to build around them, with the minimum of fuss. Quite calmly, they tell themselves (in amongst the clamour of everybody else saying the same thing), 'It'll happen. All those years of trying not to, and now we're jamming the gears into reverse and expecting it to kick in right away! There's nothing wrong here. Give those little fellas a chance!'

I remember, a good fifteen months into the give it a chance period, my father's kind wish that the holiday we had coming up – two blissful weeks on a Greek island – was just what the doctor ordered. I knew what he was talking about. Tuck yourself away in a cosy holiday nest; get with the sun and the sea, with each other; let nature do the talking. And the kind sparkle that was in his eye, of course, was the one that he wanted to see reflected in ours, the one he knew we were looking for ourselves. He still believed it would happen – naturally. And we did too, certainly for a couple of hazy, blindfolded years. Why? Because it's so difficult to think of the story being written any other way: rip up the bloody script just when you've got hold of it, so soon into playing the best two parts you've ever had. So you don't. You tell yourself that it will happen, all in good time.

L was known to her friends and family for years as being a woman who loved children. A godmother ten times over! The woman without fail to remember a birthday; turn up trumps at Christmas. What a natural mother she'd make. Plus, she has Mediterranean blood coursing through her veins. Her father's mother was from Seville, and his father's family was a mix of Spanish, Italian and Greek. Wherever she goes across that band of warm countries, people take her as one of their own (she has a beautifully strong, southern Mediterranean face, olive sun-ready skin, dark eyes framed by dark hair). Her father had three sisters, and one of them had eight daughters. So the culture of children flows in her blood. But here she was, stalling at the threshold. What pressure.

So the haze period rolls on. The body blow to self-esteem that taking off the blindfold would inflict is too much to bear. A strike to the heart of gender, and human purpose, too, for that matter. Quite simply, what was L's main role at this stage of her life, if not this, this middle eight of mother and baby? Unthinkable. Except when you have no choice, when you're awake at three in the morning and some dark panic bird of thought is struggling free, despite your kicking and screaming to get back to sleep. 'Oh Christ. I'm infertile. No baby. No me. Nothing.' And whilst men are often at the very sharp end of infertility[1], from what I saw L go through, and several others since, it's women who find the situation (even) more unbearable, and have so much at stake at this crunch time of their lives.

The final chapter of the haze period began when we opted to check out a natural fertility clinic[2], in a leafy north London suburb. We met after work on a fine May evening, in a handsome street lined with trees pinching out their new, bright green leaves. A couple we knew whizzed past on their scooter, slowing to wave at us and shout 'Ciao bella' above their Vespa din. The rite of spring itself. Rather obviously, the main talk at the Natural Fertility Clinic was all about doing it naturally, giving yourselves the best possible chance of conceiving, at home, under relatively normal conditions, rather than those imposed by science in hospital-like surrounds. Carefully explained in holistically scientific terms, L was shown how to watch and measure the 'biological markers' of her fertility cycle in a precise way; to become her very own expert on her body's ability to conceive. Natural Procreative Technology is the method. And once a cycle or two have been monitored, a problem – sometimes missed in more conventional gynaecology – can be identified and addressed (for example, odd bleeding patterns, or insufficient cervical mucus flow). For most couples practising natural fertility, the real change this introduces to daily life is the monitoring of a woman's temperature around her ovulation. Exactly when, L learned to measure, was the right time for her to have sex. All well and good. But you need to be up for the chase! Even if it means tearing across town to be there, ready for action.

A friend of mine has a nice chase story. He and his wife already had one baby, but a serious illness meant their plans for a second were in jeopardy. Naturally, she was worried sick and was desperate to make it happen. 'Get ready,' she warned him. 'Always expect the call!' A few months later, he was overseas on a work trip, sitting in an edit suite, viewing his previous day's filming. He got a call. 'Hello, Darling,' he said, cheerily noting his wife's UK mobile number. 'Hi. I'm ovulating,' came the reply. 'Right, well I'm in Southern Italy,

3

and you're in London,' he replied, quietly and a little defensively. 'No, I'm not. I'm in your hotel room,' came her firm response. 'See you in five minutes!'

Certainly, all the attention on natural feels good. You still believe a baby is going to come naturally, and focussing on the nature of sex endorses this belief. I liked the sense of empowerment it gave us, and looking back, it was a wholesome precursor to what was to follow, in the form of more interventionist fertility treatment. In many ways, we were ticking the natural boxes anyway – being careful about what we ate, about what we drank, about having sex at the right times (afternoon is a good bet, apparently), even propping up L's legs afterwards, draining it all up as far as it would go. I don't recall having sex on the Cerne Abbas Giant (on his proud member, to be more specific), nor any other ancient fertility spots, but we certainly went the distance. But it does take time, as all holistic approaches do, a real investment of several months, at least. And, as was just beginning to dawn on us, we didn't have much time.

The second time we visited the Natural Fertility Clinic, to check on how we were doing (not great, obviously), we left in just as upbeat a fashion as after our first visit, a couple of months earlier. Not least because we were going to a couple's house for dinner, half a mile's walk away, old and good friends of L's. A couple, as it happened, who were six to eight months ahead of us in their efforts to conceiving a child, just about to embark on their first round of full IVF. I remember the look of concern on their faces when we told them where we were at, a stage that they clearly considered to be hardly out of the blocks. They even suggested, bluntly I thought at the time, that we cut to the chase, find an IVF clinic and catch them up. But we didn't want to hear them. Not yet. And this is a crucial point: whatever stage we were at in dealing with our infertility, only we – the two of us together, preferably – could decide when it was time to move on. No one else can push you along, not before you're good and ready to tackle what might be next: natural fertility; IVF; donor egg; donor sperm; no to children; adoption; surrogacy. Whichever it is. Stage by careful stage.

Around this time, we also checked out the basics of adoption. We booked ourselves on two sessions, the first to find out about intercountry adoption, the second to get an idea of what was involved in domestic adoption. The overseas session was a one-day workshop, organised by The Intercountry Adoption Centre[3], in north London. It was a fun day, run by pragmatic enthusiasts and attended by a lively group. The morning was mostly talks about the kinds of journeys we could expect should we decide to proceed: the similarities and differences between different countries, the workings of The

Hague Convention[4], ratified by an increasing number of countries to protect the human rights of children.

After a stroll and a snack in the park, we spent the afternoon playing an intercountry board game. Each couple was assigned a different country from those that are workable destinations for UK prospective adopters – Russia, China, Guatemala, Vietnam, India, etc. As we rolled our dice, we progressed or retreated around the board, experiencing some of the standard joys and frustrations of adopting from our country (I think we chose Guatemala). One roll instructed us to return home, pinged for incomplete paper work. Another ordered us to wait in country for 12 weeks. And much, much worse to consider was the news that our child's visa had been refused. Other cards were more joyous: you've been matched, proceed to country, or placement approved. It was just a game at this stage, a little food for thought.

Next up was an introductory session with Hounslow, our local borough, concerning domestic adoption. No board games to lighten the load, this time. The adoption team – bright, sensitive and calm – took us carefully through the process: home study; approval by panel; matching and placement; finalisation.

Some weeks later, I found myself talking to my mother about our adoption sessions. We could, I suggested confidently, wrap our lives around an adopted child. But I'm not sure if that was true, back then. L found the Be My Baby publication that was passed around the room quite traumatic. We both did, and for several weeks we were haunted by some of those children's faces beaming out of the magazine, some as young as one, some as old as ten, some on their own, some as sibling groups. It was nothing to do with adoption itself. We knew that to be as old and as good as the hills. But at this too early stage, we were charged by the emotional impact of these heart-breaking pictures, not by the more rational possibilities of adoption as a way forward, for us. Ironically, we couldn't see past the children.

Meanwhile, back at the coalface of our lives, we were nearly two years into it not happening. We weren't going to adopt. And the truth was that we were getting nowhere; that all the monthly hoping for the best, the fastidious checking of temperatures, and the crazy dashes across town, probably weren't going to make the difference. The facts of the matter were beginning to stare us in the face.

So, just three years into our marriage, we woke up to the fact that it was time to rip up the script – that hand-me-down script that went 'Just relax, let it happen, let nature take its course.' And some awakening it proved to be.

2
Bear traps

There are no schedules to infertility, no route maps, and no one else is showing you the way. And even if they were, you most likely wouldn't be ready to see which way they were pointing, or hear what they had to say. The next couple of years, prior to our first cycle of IVF, were for us (and I suspect for many couples) perhaps the most difficult down the infertility road. Throughout this period, we woke up to what was happening and although we began to get to grips with it, we found ourselves more rudderless than either of us had ever thought possible.

For most of us, losing control is, at the very least, alarming. And it was this loss of control over our natural desires and abilities to start a family that came to haunt us, month after month. It comes in many forms. The world that you have grown to accept and become accustomed to suddenly changes and the roles you expected to play lose their bearings. This, I think, is what derails so many people, singles or couples, as they try to steer a way through it. It's fear too, fear of what the ramifications of infertility might be – childlessness, failure, and ultimately perhaps, splitting up. Stronger couples than us, I remember thinking, weren't surviving the rigours, sadness and loss encountered throughout their infertility. Here's how one couple fell into some of those traps. Most of them took us by stealth, and they can open up beneath your feet at any stage of the journey.

Let's start with a big one, and the hardest surely, to talk about, certainly for men. Sex. One of *the* defining aspects and key measures we have of a long-term relationship. Anyone who's been together a while knows that sex changes –

boils off, simmers, cools. It's a gradual, mostly declining shift; a kick in the teeth even under the most fecund, natural course of events imaginable, particularly in those first years of life-bending, new parenthood. But infertility, and the treatments we choose to help us through it, can knock our sexual lives off track like nothing else (well before any compensatory joys of new parenthood). When a friend of mine, two years down the IVF track with his girlfriend, heard that we were lining up for treatment ourselves, his main advice was 'Look after your sex life. Guard it with your lives!' Good advice. But doomed. And given, of course, on the back of his own having taken a sensitive blow.

Sex for sheer pleasure, for its lovely now and again kick that connects us so strongly to our relationship, and to the core of ourselves. This is the most powerful aspect of our sexual lives to take a hit. All couples trying for a child experience a change to their sex lives, to some degree, even if it simply means stopping birth control and trying a bit harder to hit the monthly beats. But for couples battling infertility, sex can become shockingly functional, something so much other than the instinctive and pleasurable act of itself. When you need to produce to order, then there's a whole different agenda going on, one more akin to work time, not bedtime. Quite literally, sometimes, the kind of infertility sex you get used to goes against the grain. Production of best sperm, eggs, vaginal environment, etc. All to order. Fast, regular and same same. Like a short order chef. I have yet to hear another, more positive version from anyone who has been through it.

When L and I met, we warmed up to sex quite slowly, over several months. She was heading out of a long relationship, needing to know it was over and something new and meaningful had begun. I was quite happy to wait, happy with what I was falling into. When the flag came down, there followed a precious few years either side of our marriage when the emotional and physical states of our union joined at the hip and roamed blissfully free. It was a fearless and uninhibited time, and for the first time of my adult life, I felt not just the strong sense of arrival, but also the sweeter sense of the future. I mention this because now I can see just how far we had to fall. It was a steep, dangerous drop from those lush, high pastures of our first few years. It is for any of us. And how we fell, L and I, discovering the hammerblows of infertility through an act that had been so much *ours*, one that was now failing to provide us with that next, natural state. It was as if someone had broken in and ripped out the precious, sexual core of our lives, dragged it away, kicking and screaming. And it's very, very shocking to find yourself being let down so ungently. It seems the most unnatural thing in the world.

Throughout infertility, we hear some memorably crass and insensitive remarks. That's a given. People don't mean it, and there's plenty who show the care and forethought not to follow suit, bless them. And undoubtedly it's a very sensitive time – of course we can find ourselves overreacting to a scenario that otherwise we might sail through. But I found sex to be the zone most vulnerable to a thoughtlessly lobbed grenade. Here, I'm sure, is quite a common example. I was out one evening, meeting a guy who was going to brief me on a substantial piece of TV production work. He had his girlfriend with him. Both had been previously married with children, now freshly separated and blushingly keen on each other. Suffice to say in a very different place to me (this sense of feeling outside the regular loop, emotionally as well as physically, is a regular one amongst infertility people). Well, whilst the guy was at the bar, his girlfriend asked me whether I had kids. I told her I didn't, and then she wanted to know why not, at my age? Christ, if there's one golden rule this whole trip has branded me with, it is never, repeat never, to enquire as to whether anyone has kids or not! Kids reveal themselves soon enough in a person's life, if the answer's not blindingly obvious already. Anyway, as sometimes happens, and without meaning to, I found myself giving a very straight answer to this woman, a total stranger, one I would most likely never see again. I told her that I was married, that we both wanted children, but that it wasn't happening for us. 'Ah, what a shame,' she replied, adding with a chirpy kind of a nudge and a wink, 'Still, at least it's good fun trying!' She was nice enough, meant nothing really, by her remark. But I found myself boiling over with anger. Very nearly in tears and going white at the knuckles, I could have punched her lights out. Not surprisingly, our get-together didn't continue much further into the night (even though I did manage to land the work).

All this talk of sex brings me to an additional, thorny scenario L and I had to deal with, even before we had any kind of grip on our infertility. Very ironically, coming off the pill meant sex became painful for L. Not always, but often enough. She had a surprisingly common condition called endometriosis[1], and one of the positive side effects of the pill was that it masked the symptoms and pain of the condition. Endometriosis is a strange thing to try and visualize. It occurs when small gluey bits of womb lining tissue are found growing in the wrong place, outside of the uterus. The tissue goes on responding to a monthly hormone cycle, meaning it bleeds. But the blood can't escape, and this causes lesions, or cysts – areas of painful inflammation found right across the pelvic area (commonly on ovaries). And since the pill masks so much of the natural period, it can, as in L's case, only come to light once a woman stops taking it. Surprisingly little is known about endometriosis and its cause. Suffice to say it's a major cause of stress, pain and anxiety for many women. Commonly, pain and discomfort are worse around ovulation. So just at the time when you should be feeling super-fertile and ready, you most often don't, you just feel exhausted or, worse still, quite ill. And just at the time when you should be up for it, guess what, penetrative sex can hurt like hell.

Endometriosis is treatable, or at least some of the resulting lesions and soreness are treatable (there's more lasting help, too, to be had from nutritionists). And it needs treating (or bypassing) since it can, itself, be a cause of infertility. A laparoscopy can locate the outcast bits of frayed, damaged tissue, which then can be cut away, through a keyhole incision close to the navel. L had two of these procedures, to try and ease her discomfort, and eradicate the possibility of endometriosis being a suspect cause of infertility. When I picked her up from the London Women's Clinic[2], after her second treatment for endometriosis, I remember the friendly duty nurse saying to me, 'All clear now, darlin', nothing to stop your wife having her baby!' And of course, I took her gift of hope, wanted to leave the hospital buoyed up by her optimism, carry it back into our lives. You learn to look for every scrap of hope you can.

To this day, I can't say that I have fully dealt with the loss around our sex lives that we experienced throughout this time. And I don't know whether any amount of therapy would have helped me mourn its going, across all these years. I know just how acutely L experienced that loss, too. At worst, it causes a couple to leave each other. It's too painful. At best, over time, you find ways of putting some of the pieces back together.

I found talking with L about the loss of what seemed like a whole chunk of my life the hardest thing to do. Talking about it only deepened the disappointment of its going, made it more *real*. So I didn't. I kept my self-serving sadness mostly to myself, shielded the shame of its going as much as its actual loss by imagining it wasn't there. And not surprisingly, the more I kept quiet, the more my spirits sank.

L's sadness was anchored more around the loss of her fertility. Yes, that physical blow to our relationship was very significant for her, too. But at the heart of her *going quiet* was an inability to articulate the intensity of her feelings around her infertility and all it meant (including the nagging, sometimes intense sense of dysfunction and failure). If my inability to communicate my loss was about the present, perhaps hers was more about the future, about what she knew would be denied to her in years to come. And what a blank, barren future she could see. No wonder she didn't want to dissect it all, particularly with me, her co-conspirator in this whole numbing affair. No wonder, just like I did, she pretended it wasn't there, constructed an easier and different kind of present around other people, or too much time at work – compensatory ploys that buried the longing under something else.

Short of abusive behaviour, I can't think there's much else more destructive to the inner sanctum of a relationship than two people staying schtum and hoping a bombshell like infertility will go away. But no amount of anyone telling me this at the time would have made a bean of a difference. You know it makes sense to talk. You know that the lack of tackling infertility together, openly, is the very thing that is screwing you up. But you don't. At least, not fully. Even if you've had all the counselling in the world. You can't plan for it, as with everything else that infertility flings at you. You just have to hope that knowing about it gives you an edge, at least in retrospect, if and when you can talk about it later, with the benefit of all that experience.

I remember one Saturday morning when our communication levels hit rock bottom. We were both full of work and both stuck in our sadness. A free weekend opened its arms ahead of us, a whole life-saving raft of opportunities to talk. But we couldn't take it. I sat at the top of the stairs, listening to L showering and then cleaning her teeth. I don't think we had any plans, maybe a Sainsbury's run for one of us. This was the kind of weekend that a couple of years earlier we'd have lapped up and loved. But we didn't understand what we were dealing with, and what we could follow we lacked the wherewithal to talk about. We made tea and breakfast. Then nothing. Nothing except the raw, radio silence of our infertility. L broke out first. She went back upstairs and got ready to go out. I followed her and sat on the stairs again. Neither of us could slow or speed or cut the mood. We had shared so much, given each other so much in common. And now this between us, this aching, muted discovery. She was crying as she went down the stairs and turned up to look at me when she reached the door. Any other circumstances – critical illness, a death in the family, a firing from work – would have turned the moment on its head that morning, would have had us pause, batten down the hatches on our silence and find each other's outstretched arms. But not this, this foul infertility thing.

Throughout most of this time, L had the help of individual counselling and was used to its restorative force. But we didn't have counselling as a couple, and I can now see that this was a mistake. We could have done with somebody to help us explore how we felt about these complicated, stressful processes; explore our feelings around our worth, our disappointment and our failings.

To offer a wider view on our sadness and help us join it all up. Today, most IVF clinics can put you in touch with a counsellor, should you want one. Some of them have even been through it themselves.

A constant throughout our infertility, I can now see, is that when we needed to be most strongly supportive of each other – all those endless monthly let-downs, IVF cycles, test after bloody test – we were just as likely to find ourselves moving apart. Some of this, I'm sure, is the gender gap rearing its uglier head, a kind of instinctive lack of emotional understanding, or knowledge, between men and women. Just when you need to be your best as a team, you can find yourself turning away, driven by an alarming lack of emotional sync.

Here's one shameful example. L was bed-resting near the end of her first cycle of IVF, giving her embryos their best chance of hatching out. I was home from work soon after lunch, to help out, do some chores, generally lighten L's load. These are tense, tired times, the final few days before the first blood test to see what, if anything, has happened. The best you can do is lie back, get lost in a good book or a movie, and hope. Hence the looking after bit. It started fine: a pile of washing, clearing up, cooking. Then upstairs to see if L wanted anything. She did. It was teatime and she could've murdered a cuppa. 'One small hitch,' she said. 'We're out of milk.' Well, you'd think that'd be easy enough. Pop out for some cow juice, whizz back home and fix the tea. But no. Some small but significant link in the short leash I was on pulled up short and snapped. 'Fuck that,' I thought. 'I could have picked up milk at any number of stores on my way home, and much more than that, this whole bloody show is all about you. Me? A sideshow, a runner, at best, sperm beaker in one hand, over-loaded life plate in the other.' Of course, I didn't communicate it quite like that. Nothing that bold and open. And anyway, I didn't need to. L knew exactly what was going on. Five minutes later, of course, I was full of pathetic remorse, whining on about compassion fatigue like it meant anything.

Such outlets of steam are awkward to explain, harder to deal with and forgive. More of a man thing, perhaps: I have reacted like that since, and will again I expect, around other scenarios. God knows we can feel the closeness of our relationship slipping away from us, even in the best of times. But in difficult periods the risk is only increased. What you know as caring, thoughtful and sensitive can sharpen their edges into more dangerous tools…So expect some madness along the way. You *will* see it! And when you do, if you possibly can, cut it some appropriate slack.

Of course, the times when you hurtle off the tracks are easier to understand when you're more safely back on them. We were fortunate, I think, to make it through this period. What we needed most was a clear memory of the relationship we began. We had this, L and I, and we never lost sight of it completely, at least not for too long. It worked as a kind of base camp, a safe place to return to and from which to try the next assault.

And here's the positive amongst the pitfalls, a very hard fought, hard won positive. At the heart of all this uncharted and rudderless experience can be the discovery of what the two can bring to each other. You have to look out for each other; learn more about the other's condition – all of their conditions. Yes, infertility can break you down, break you up even. But what it can also give you, deeply and slowly learned, will endure.

3
The helping hand of science

There was no doubt that we were ready to venture out into the world of reproductive science. Several London clinics were immediately on our radars, but the one that came most recommended was ARGC, Assisted Reproduction & Gynaecology Centre[1], run by one of the UK's most successful and best known fertility experts, Dr Mohammed Taranissi[2]. We knew two couples who'd had quite different but equally positive experiences to share with us. Both had successfully conceived there, and we had met their children to show for it. It sounds a little evangelical, but you need to *believe* in the place and its people, and a trusted recommendation can endorse the decision you make like nothing else. Just to be sure, we went to check out a couple of other options – none of these courses of action are determined overnight.

One of those was Dr Geeta Nargund, now Director of Create Health Clinics[3], about whom we had heard great things (a fountain of knowledge on all things infertility). She was then Head of the Centre for Reproductive Medicine at St George's, in Tooting, South London. Her speciality is natural and mild assisted reproduction techniques, with minimum or zero use of drugs. Conventional IVF uses powerful drugs to force an artificial cycle then stimulate the ovaries to produce several eggs. Dr Nargund's 'soft IVF'[4] uses hormone stimulation during a woman's normal cycle, and less powerful drugs. Overall, we knew that success rates weren't as high as with conventional IVF, but it sounded good and we were keen to find out more.

Dr Nargund[5] was an inspiring, galvanizing person to meet. Efficiently and nicely, she got to her point. What we needed, in our case, despite our shared natural concerns around the drugs, was fully stimulated IVF. And she made it perfectly clear that we needed to get a move on. Why? The evidence was stacking up against us: no pregnancies; the wrong side of forty; endometriosis.

To make her point, she told us something that has always stayed with me. Even when a couple get it together at the very peak of their reproductive curve – when their egg and sperm quality are second to none – there is still, at very best, only a 50% chance of conception. Extraordinary that so many of us are here at all! Furthermore, she told us, a woman's quality and quantity of egg production begins to diminish earlier than had previously been thought – considerably sooner into her thirties or even her late 20s, depending on several factors. There is, she explained, a whole mythology grown up around the notion of women being able to conceive later in their reproductive lives, through IVF. The headlines that catch our eye – IVF mums well into their 40s – become accepted as the cultural norm. But the reality is that the success rates drop off sharply. The younger you are, the more chance you have, and even then, it's quite low. We needed to understand that our window of opportunity was already beginning to close.

Sobering stuff. We left Tooting that afternoon in a hurry, totally dispossessed, as if we needed any further dispossession, of any fertility thoughts unconnected to full-on IVF. The next day L rang ARGC and signed us up. Quite suddenly, we had a plan. Signing up for IVF, although we knew our chances were way less than 50/50, felt like a blast of fresh air. It was a relief to now feel that we were taking action; that we were, in some limited way, regaining control. Following soon after, our first meeting at ARGC spurred us on. Confidence in the team is vital, and Taranissi instilled lots of it in the thorough and open way he went about assessing our best chances of success. When he wasn't studying our notes, or peering at scans, he looked us in the eye and included us in his plans, progress and problems. Managing expectations around fertility treatment is near impossible, but in his low-key, positive way, he certainly tried to keep our feet on the ground.

Away from the clinic, it was equally encouraging to read about ARGC's success rates, around twice the national average, across the age range. All fertility clinics, NHS[6] and private, advertise their success rates in their brochures and on their websites. And not surprisingly, a kind of a league table has grown up over the past decade (at the top of which are the private clinics), where positioning is determined solely by success rates – meaning, to use the same blunt language as they do, the number of IVF births, *live* births. That's what counts, after all, for us and them. It was also around this time that I first came across the Human Fertilisation Embryology Authority, known as HFEA[7], an excellent source of news and information on all UK fertility issues, including clinics, their comparative success rates (accompanied by a well-worded warning note around the perils of following the league) and their prices.

Signed up and raring to go, L discovered she had another wait in store, before she could start her first cycle of IVF. The cause of the holdup was her follicle-stimulating hormone levels[8], measured as being too high. FSH levels are a pretty good indicator of a woman's egg quantity and to a lesser extent, quality (egg quality is still the most difficult factor to determine in the whole infertility treatment process). An FSH measure of below eight suggests a positive amount and quality of eggs. If it's higher, then it points to the likelihood that the pituitary gland, which controls FSH levels, is over stretching itself to produce eggs (more and more likely as a woman's egg reserve starts to decline). So, wanting to maximize the chances of a successful IVF cycle, ARGC don't go ahead. And with good reason, when you consider what's involved, emotionally and financially. We understood the rationale, and valued the ethics, but here was yet another round of monthly disappointments.

Two things eased this period of frustrating waits. Firstly, L concentrated on getting herself in the best possible health, fertility wise. She'd heard about and went to see a fertility expert called Zita West[9], and thought she was terrific. With her open-minded and holistic approach to fertility, Zita is well known for helping prepare women and men for cycles of IVF, improving their health to maximize their chances of success. Key issues include nutrition, stress, emotional and physical support, overall wellbeing and the right kind of positive mindset. She begins with an IVF Support Consultation and then draws up a personal plan of approach for each woman or couple. (Today, she has her own well established and independent fertility clinic, offering a wide range of fertility treatment pathways.) Most helpful, L found, was the acupuncture sessions Zita recommended, both before and after implantation. Her faith in needles has been endorsed by mounting evidence[10] that acupuncture increases blood flow to the uterus, so thickening and regulating the uterine lining, and improving the chances of good embryo implantation.

Secondly, we got a dog. A wonderful, complicated, alpha female pup called Jess. Yes, alright! Of course she was a child substitute! But what the hell. We needed something to give; to start rocking the boat. Something else to love and shout at besides ourselves. I knew it didn't make much sense. I was about to start a new job and L about to kick into IVF, bed rest and all. But I went along with it, and everything that having a dog entails. Not surprisingly, right from the off, attachment and bonding were strong (at least from our side of the basket).

Well, the spirit-lifting combination of acupuncture and Jessie dog did the trick. Within weeks of her arrival, L's FSH levels had dropped sufficiently for ARGC to start us on our first cycle of IVF. We were up and running, ready for whatever our date with medical science was going to throw at us.

Apart from all the scans (to check for example, the condition of the uterus wall), the blood tests, the consultations (before, during and after), and the drugs of course, here's what a cycle of IVF is, in a technical nutshell – what actually happens to a woman at ARGC and all IVF clinics up and down the land. In vitro fertilization (the in vitro bit is from the Latin inside the glass, as opposed to in vivo, meaning in the living body) involves four clear stages. First, the stimulation (with hormonal drugs) of her ovulation process, more precisely the stimulation of multiple follicles of her ovaries, so producing, ideally, more eggs than in a usual cycle. Second, the removal, usually called retrieval, of her eggs (Latin name ova). Third, the fertilization of these eggs with sperm, in a liquid. And fourth, the transfer of fertilized, cell-divided eggs to her uterus (Latin zygote at a three-day stage, or blastocyst at five days) in the hope that one of them will successfully implant and grow.

Ovum, zygote, blastocyst. What beautiful language! Not of this world, somehow, but rather from a Spock to Captain Kirk exchange, or some incredible sci-fi detail from 'Fantastic Voyage'. I loved it, this knowing a new process, these new, life force words. Words that other people, the doing-what-comes-naturally gang, most likely weren't party to. It felt special and the science felt good.

All well and good. Now here's what happens, sooner or later, to most blokes (when they're not fretting over their partner's health or their rising IVF bills). Some of the clinics I have looked at online have a video tour of the facilities. About half way through a smiling nurse directs a wholesome looking chap into a small room. This is the sample room (called a masterbetorium in some clinics!), so the soothing voice-over tells us, as the nurse closes the door and leaves him to his fate. It's time to look inside the sample room, see what goes on. Once inside, there's usually a chair, just one, and a table. On the table is a neat spread of porn mags (very 1970s!) although these days I gather there are more digital options (a friend of mine whose sperm issues saw him visiting dozens of sample rooms told me that he became preoccupied with a porn-search defined by its beautiful photography, something far more stylish than the usual glamour!). There now ensues a curious otherworldly kind of few moments. You can hear staff pottering about on the other side of the door. The next guy is lined up in the waiting room, knowing what's expected of him, but wondering if he's going to be up to the job. Your partner, bless her, is having some scan or blood test downstairs. And you're bent over a Penthouse, trying to snake charm a few million of your finest swimmers into a small plastic beaker. Still, as the nice woman in the bar reminded me, at least it's good fun trying.

Here's a diary entry from one of those encounters: *L downstairs, heavily sedated, having her eggs collected, ready for pick 'n' mix later in the week. Me? Just jerked off in a little plastic jar with my name on it, as usual. Had a quick look at one of the mags. Well thumbed. Must remember to tell them to freshen up the stocks when I sign the guest book. Ended up checking out a few small ads (why not when you've got the chance?). Amongst all the phone ads, this one caught my eye…PREGNANT PHONE SEX! And there she was, a vastly pregnant woman advertising herself in her bra and suspenders. Underneath she exclaimed PREGNANT & HORNY!*

I have talked to a number of men about the pleasures of IVF sample rooms over the years (the joys of research). I guess there are other, more emotionally intelligent ways of connecting with men who have been down the IVF route. But you know how guys are, and it's always been a good icebreaker for me. One work friend of mine has a story I'm particularly fond of, and he is kind enough to let me tell it here. Throughout IVF, he told me, he found the rigors of the sample room overbearingly intimidating. Quite simply, he couldn't perform. On the first of these unfortunate occasions – after sweating out the initial panic – he had the bright idea of phoning his girlfriend, who was sitting in the waiting room. Brilliant! Answering his call, she left the waiting room, gave the appropriate number of quiet knocks on the sample room door and snuck in. For my friend, help was at hand and moments later, he duly presented his brimming beaker to the nurse. And so it was on the second and third occasions his sperm was called upon. But on the fourth occasion, events took a different, more adventurous turn. His partner called him from work, and quite unexpectedly, told him he needed to get up to town, pronto, and deliver a sample. 'Fine,' he said, expecting her to meet him there in a couple of hours, create a little scene in the sample room, maybe a light lunch afterwards. 'Impossible,' she said. 'Piled high with work and can't get out. You'll have to be a big boy and do it yourself. And get on with it!' Trembling with responsibility, he found himself later that afternoon locking the sample room door behind him. He didn't even try and warm up, knew he didn't have a hope in hell of doing a job. So, clutching the small plastic beaker with his name on it, he dashed out of the building, wildly forming his plan as he dashed. There it was, just across the street, a Travel Lodge! Heaven, he thought, as he belted over. Some privacy. A little TV perhaps, maybe even a lie down. Suddenly it all seemed possible. He booked himself in, for a one-hour slot. Naturally, the woman on reception was rather curious as to the purpose of his visit. And so he found himself telling her his IVF woes, pointing rather madly in the direction of the clinic and the grim confines of its sample room. 'Oh,' she said. 'Poor you, how awful for you! Of course you can have a room for an hour. How brave of you both!' The rest was straight forward, by comparison. Forty minutes later – showered and trouser-pressed – he was skipping lightly down the stairs, his warm and safely capped beaker in his pocket. Ah yes, he thought, the small matter of checking out. Thank God – the same woman on reception. 'How did you get on Sir, find everything you needed?' She enquired, brightly. 'Pretty good, thanks, er….Jenny,' he cheerfully replied, as he studied the name badge on her chest and patted his pocket. 'Oh, good, Sir! I'm so pleased we could help.' By this time, my friend had produced his wallet, and was reaching for his Visa card. But she stopped him in his tracks. 'No, no, Sir! Not for such a short time, not for such a good cause!' He thanked her a little more than he might have done under more usual circumstances, said his goodbyes, and sauntered back to the clinic, mighty relieved and with a new take on 'one on the house'. You will be pleased to hear, I'm sure, that he is now a proud father. (And a better advert for Travel Lodge I'm yet to see.)

One more story from the sample room collection, this one from friends of friends. The couple concerned duly showed up at their London clinic on the morning of egg retrieval. They checked in and she headed off to the lab. In due course, he was handed his beaker and escorted to the sample room. Unlike the previous guy, he got to it and pdq had produced his sample. Top firmly back on, label checked. All good. Now in this lab, there's a wonderfully low-tech post room system for delivering sperm samples to the lower floor lab. You pop the beaker into an opening, and then, as if in a Cohen Brothers film, it glides invisibly down a chute before making a nice soft landing in the lab below. From there it's in the safe hands of the experts. This our hero did, before retreating to the waiting room, as instructed. Thirty minutes passed, then several more. 'Strange,' he thought. 'Should've been called down by now. Must be a hold up.' Then the nurse who had shown him the sample room happened to pass the waiting room, and noticed him twiddling his thumbs. 'All OK?' she enquired. 'Yup, all fine, posted the sample nearly an hour ago,' he replied. Her face paled. Doh! Our hero's sample, it transpired, had got itself wedged somewhere in the chute. So off they went to the maintenance room, down in the basement, where the boys in overalls were enjoying a tea break. Not for long. Soon they were fighting the fire, lifting ceiling panels and floor boards in a spirited attempt to locate the wedged beaker. Which eventually they did, a couple of hours later. All safe and sound on the sperm front. Except of course, it was too late for the freshly retrieved batch of eggs. 'Bugger!' Our man had no option but to go again. So he was ushered back upstairs and shown the sample room. Once more with feeling. Top securely on. Check the name. And off it went, except this time, he delivered it himself, carefully taking the stairs.

The ground floor at ARGC was a busy, flustered kind of place, run by Ellie (at least it was then), Mr T's wife, and her team of flat out administrators. Sometimes flustered became brusque, although understandable, to a degree, when you consider the frontline nature of the work, and the level of emotions coming in off the street. Front of house is where IVF catches up with you, where it can boil over, where suddenly it's real. It's where you do the waiting, the nail biting; where FSH levels were patiently explained to me by Ellie, after L was told for the third consecutive month that she couldn't start a cycle; where you wait for your hormone drugs and a session on how to use them, or your first egg retrieval, or your follow-up meeting with Taranissi after it didn't work out. It's where you check out other women and couples waiting for various bits of their process, too, find yourself wondering what their chances are, up against yours. Perhaps that woman over there is someone you've seen online, maybe chatted to about clinics, protocols, what happened, what didn't. This is the place where you feverishly get to scratch that bloody great itch. Same in any clinic up and down the land, surely.

Yes, I saw emotions run high at ARGC. It's babies we're here for, after all, not a tooth check-up. Plus, you're surrounded by pictures of IVF success. Pictures of smiling, bouncing babies, crowding the walls of the hallway and Ellie's admin office. A great montage mush of mums and babies. And thank you notes, to Mr T and the gang, covered in crosses. Sickening! I knew why they were there, to encourage us all; fuel the dream. But I remember thinking that this wasn't helping me at all. That I wouldn't need much of a prompt to pull the whole bloody lot down. Just like all those kid pictures people at work stick on the edge of their PC screens make you feel, only much worse. (Apologies if this is just me. I guess it's never too late for those anger sessions.)

Beware of those waiting rooms (in my experience, and I'm sure for most men with frontline experience). Nowhere is your sidelined role (so it seems) more keenly felt than in the waiting rooms and corridors of fertility clinics, labs and hospitals. Even if the infertility is *yours*, it's you who's doing most of the waiting. Waiting rooms are exactly what they say they are – rooms where you *wait*, where time and purpose get stuck in the most awkward way, and where, if you're there for long enough, you start to uncoil enough rope of doom and gloom to hang yourself. A fug creeps in, a toxic takeover by anxiety, guilt, money worries, loss of masculinity, purpose and direction... 'Why me? Why us?'

But downstairs, down in the basement. Ah! Here's where the beauty of science holds your hand, takes a grip of your spirit and glides you through. It's a quiet, serene place: everybody wearing muted, light blue trousers and smock tops, going about their ultra-serious business in a purposeful, hushed manner. That's the kind of calm vibe you want from an IVF lab. And a reassuring sense of precision and skill, not simply around their science, but in the respectful way they met our wide-eyed questions. Here's where I fell for IVF, down here in the lab, a place of science and mystery, of reality and hope, with the fragility of life's extraordinary start, quite literally, under the microscope.

There are two clips from that first IVF memory bank that I shall always hold dear. The first is when we were called into the lab to see our three-day old fertilised eggs (embryos already!), our zygotes. L's stimulated cycle had produced five good quality eggs (as far as they could tell) from a total of eight. Two were now selected for freezing, stored away for another day. And here we were, in the warm underground lull of the lab, holding our breath and peering down a microscope at the remaining three, the three that in a couple of days would be transferred to their rightful place, L's womb. Brave first circles of life! We were full of questions, but speechless in the presence of these spheres, these lovely craters of cell divisions, moon-like, gently held within the egg's watery circumference. Is this how NASA technicians felt, I wondered, when they first saw that satellite image of our round and beautifully patched earth, flickering onto their screens?

Once back outside, with the hairs on the back of our necks nearer their normal lie, we were quietly buzzing on the privilege of being able to witness the possible beginnings of new life like this. *Our* new lives, so it seemed, inscribed in these tiny eggs. Years later, I still see their rounded forms – the rings from a rising fish, or from rain, or when I'm driving at night, and the round, watery tail lights of cars up ahead focus into view.

The second one? A couple of days later, when Mr T transferred those three fertilized eggs back into the middle lining of L's womb. Not surprisingly, she was lying down, everything important accessible. I was sitting beside her, watching, and in a few minutes, utterly transported. One of his lab assistants had loaded a catheter with our eggs and I remember Taranissi holding it aloft as he got comfortable and steady in his chair, adjusting his thick glasses one last time. He had a screen to check, a fuzzy, video-noisy image from abdominal ultrasound, so he could track the catheter tip's progress, through the cervical opening and into the womb cavity. But he didn't seem to need it. As far I could tell, he held his breath, and with his tongue firmly between his teeth, got silently to work. Nothing else stirred in the room. And when he let them go, released them into the very core of her womb, only then did he appear to breathe out, very gently. Afterwards, the same assistant took the catheter from him, checked under the microscope that he had delivered all three. She gave him the nod. Now he looked up at L, told her he was happy with his process, advised her on bed rest to give her eggs the best possible chance to implant, and then wished her good luck. It was a masterful performance, Zen in the way it closed everything else out.

So, just before Christmas, L hit the sack for several days' bed rest. What a December gift pregnancy would be, we couldn't help telling ourselves. It's worth saying again: you find yourself ready and able to believe. You have to. But we knew how fortunate we would be for L to conceive at her first attempt. Of the several thousand women that underwent IVF treatment with their own fresh or frozen eggs that year, the UK average success rate was to be around 17%. Higher at ARGC, at around 49%. In her 39th year, we knew that her chances were, at best, fair.

Sure enough, it wasn't to be. The so-called roller coaster trip of IVF had begun. Like so many women on cycles of IVF, L had given a first positive test, only to find this 'chemical pregnancy' stage fading away after a few days' blood tests. And like so many couples desperate for a baby, within a few weeks we had moved on, ready and madly willing to try again.

4
Drumming up support

aving a decent network of strong support certainly helped us through the rigours of infertility, at the very least helped us get through the damn thing as best we could. There are all sorts of ways to go about building that support. With the risk of teaching several grandmothers how to suck eggs, here are some of them covered.

Family and friends

It's a huge help if the family are onside. That's the first thing. It's tough for the parent birds back home, wanting their grandchildren and not getting them. They, in turn, need to come to terms with it, stage by stage. But they need to get over it, stop applying any undue pressure, even if they feel it's born out of kindness, and start to build some support. This can take a while. And if it doesn't happen, then inevitably there will be rifts.

Both L and I were very fortunate in this respect. For the best part of a decade, L's mother never once laid an ounce of pressure or expectation at our door, not a scrap even, of her own inevitable sense of loss. All she wanted, in her kind and gentle way, was what was best for us. Especially for her daughter, whose suffering must have been painful for her to see. My family were strong and supportive, right from the off. For weeks, they would back off, knowing the pain and trouble it was causing us, although their support from 150 miles up the motorway was always felt. And then we would meet up and have an intensive round of sharing of how things were – tearful some of it – but handled with much sensitivity. As we arrived at each major decision point along the way, they backed us to the hilt. Indeed, we had a strong sense of our close family making the journey with us. We learned how my mother, too, had suffered from endometriosis; how she had experienced, also, that great welling of sadness and loss, when one of their proud grandparent friends, for example, hijacked another dinner party conversation with doting news and pictures of their grandchildren. In turn, they had to rip up the grandchild script, and that they did so supportively was the best thing they could do. Even if, at times, it was simply knowing when to back away and leave us to get on with it for a few weeks.

My sister was a great source of strength and support for us. She doesn't have a child, and of course this drew us together. Neither does my aunt (and for that matter, nor does L's brother, yet). There were times when we bonded over our shared experience of childlessness, lightened the mood around our combined inability to provide any next in line. Even laughed about it, sometimes.

We were fortunate too, that at different times our families contributed to the expensive process of IVF. On our final round of IVF, we badly under budgeted. I was out of work and L was taking a break. We needed some help and we got it. Knowing how the next leg of the journey is being paid for makes us so much more confident and sure around our decisions, and family money, if there's any spare, is a fine way of supporting and validating those plans you have made. After all, everyone's gunning for the same chip off the old block. They're stakeholders, too. A loan or a gift can be difficult to accept from family. But getting through infertility is usually expensive. And if they can, and are allowed to, most families want to help out.

In our experience, it was friends and not family who sometimes lacked a sensitivity around the grimmer effects of infertility we were dealing with. And perhaps this is inevitable, given the various other stages they were at, single or in the thick of having babies themselves. It's an alien task for a close friend to empathise with in any meaningful, supportive way. This is especially hard for women, whose friendships are so strongly forged, and so regularly updated several times a week. If your closest pal is pregnant, or newly mummed up, or battling with a couple of feisty toddlers, then she might just as well inhabit another planet, such is the emotional and occupational gulf between you. Even as a regular, single woman you may have lost her for a while, let alone as a woman under the coshes of infertility.

But somehow, you need to seek out the one or two friends that offer something the others don't, and coax them to keep you company. At the very least, be the sounding board that your careworn partner can't possibly (always) be. L did find strong support throughout this long period, from one or two good friends whose life circumstances allowed them the time and insight to see what was going on, to go the extra mile in their friendship. One girlfriend already had two children, both in their teens and becoming more and more independent.

She had time she could generously give to the cause. Another close friend was single during most of this time, meaning she was closely aligned and going through perhaps, some of the same pangs of wanting children herself.

Me? Men have a way of shutting down, of retreating from much of the emotional support that we so want, not to mention need. We look less hard for it amongst our friends than women do, demand less from them and have fewer expectations of them. As a result, men are more prone than women to risk the loss of their friendships. We don't take as much care over their currency. We let time and contact slip. We can be experts at that, and for much of the time, I fell into line.

In the very early stages of our IVF period, I bumped into a close friend of mine, Jon, who I'd known since day one at college. After we graduated, we moved up to London together, shared a flat and walked the streets looking for work. Now, some fifteen years later, he was living in a different part of London and married with two children. I hadn't seen him for a few months and I knew I'd let our friendship drift. He'd suffered hugely since I'd last seen him, as had his poor wife. A few months previously, he now told me, they'd lost a child, just hours after he was born. Within one monumental day, he had registered both the birth and the death of their baby. Heartbreaking.

It was early morning as we stood in the chill of that Soho street corner. We parted soon after, after he had generously thought to ask me how we were doing with our own efforts for a child. I was shocked for them both, disappointed in myself because I hadn't been around for him to have told me sooner, if he'd wanted to. But I knew then, as we parted, that as sure as his life would never be the same again, so neither would mine. The loss and grief I was experiencing around childlessness, although very different and less severe than his, would be with me always, even if, over time, the roughness of its grain would smooth. The intensity of my feelings took me by surprise that morning, as if a kind of empathy barrier had been broken through. It was, emotionally speaking, as if I'd woken up – startled by the raw tragedy of Jon's news – and found myself more capable of tackling our own circumstances of childlessness.

There were a few times, though, when I would talk for hours to a friend, as if it were quite planned. Out on a long walk perhaps, tramping over some drizzly, far-flung hill on a weekend's break. Or over a long evening's drink in a pub. A friend, most often, whose marriage or relationship was drifting close to the rocks, both of us anchoring onto that sense of edgy parity that our different circumstances brought about.

Other times, I would find myself telling a total stranger about it. Odd this, the way we can open up to people we don't know, and how adversity itself can be the thing that draws it out. Some sympathetic guy or woman I was sitting next to, on a plane perhaps, or at a dinner table. Quite unannounced, I would find myself spilling the beans, tipping out my story from the sharp edge of its tin. And yes, it brought me some support. Why? Because there's a person giving you their ear in a certain way, all the more intensely because they too understand the terms of the discourse, that just as soon as the plane lands or the evening ends, it'll be over. It's as if they can sense the gain that their listening will bring. And you can sense it too, so you go on. They allow you to clearly sound out the state you're in, as if you're listening back to yourself, slightly out of body. It's a way of placing one's perspective, or shifting it, of discovering where you're at. On the few occasions it happened to me, I found some real third party value in that.

Throughout this whole period, L gave herself an occasional licence to quietly avoid any situation that might upset her – family days with kids, maybe a wedding. God knows the emotional charge of infertility can catch you short. Just sitting near a little child on a bus can do it – just one laugh or cry or seal-eyed look, and on comes the flush. (I remember once having to stop the car for a few minutes to sort myself out before I could safely take the wheel again. I had just halted at a zebra crossing to let three primary school teachers steer a gambolling crocodile of skipping, laughing, reception-aged kids across the road. Just the sight of them had me streaming with tears and steaming up the windscreen. No warning, no announcement. Just the raw, emotional spill of what I was going through.) But sometimes, some gathering or other crops up that has red flags waving all over it. A christening; a child's birthday do; or dinner with friends who naturally enough at some point during the evening talk about their kids, even if it's just that late night nudge to their partners when it's time to go home and relieve the babysitter. These can be tough, tough assignments, and there's no shame in skipping them. I found L was much more sensitive than I was to some of these triggering occasions. She'd be fine, for hours, even at a kid's party. Then quite suddenly, she would tell me afterwards, something would strike, and she'd rapidly lose confidence amongst her peers like a busted plane losing altitude. Other times she would catch herself and we would pull out before it started, or find ourselves leaving early. The more intuitive friends knew what was happening.

Seeing the wood from the trees

A few years back, when we were going through IVF, social media wasn't the force it is today. But even then, we didn't immerse ourselves amongst the infertility or IVF chat and buzz around how, what and where we were doing – or weren't doing. L chose not to go down that path, mainly because it afforded her some distance from it all. She was scared of it dragging her in. I was more involved online, trying to ferret out the information most relevant to our own case, from the fast-growing body of online material. But we mostly kept our infertility selves to ourselves.

I remember once leaving L in the clinic and going for a coffee with a woman who we'd met a few times at the clinic, and was on much the same IVF track as us. She was, by our standards, a fountain of knowledge, albeit on an amateur level. She knew the workings of our clinic inside out, and several others, too. I think she was on her fourth or fifth cycle, and had given up work to concentrate wholly on the job of making a baby. Just as soon as we sat down and started to talk, alarm bells rang. She was, so it seemed to me (and in a totally understandable way), in too deep. I didn't have much to offer her, certainly nothing to add to her knowledge bank, and I didn't feel it was my place to try and shift her 100mph mind set. Her message to me? 'Get genned up! Get knowledgeable, know what the docs are telling you, or not telling you!' Right, of course, to some extent. But that level of single mindedness worried me.

Hard as it is, you can't let it fog you out, at least not seven days a week, to the point where you simply can't see anything else. Ferreting around online, you do get a sense of those fine lines – between rational viewpoints and the more panic-driven cries for help. When you put yourself out there – revealing your infertility hand online – you need to manage that exposure of self carefully. As supportive as our peers can undoubtedly be, it's important to protect that home base of privacy, that blockade of self-help and strength. I guess it's something that sometimes crops up in counselling sessions.

So would we be more in amongst it today, were we just about to embark on an IVF cycle at ARGC? Yes, most likely we would. It would be hard not to be, given the whole raft of stuff out there for us to roll up our sleeves and delve into. And there are some great forums and social media groups to join; one or two of them, hearteningly, started by men going through it[1], reaching out to other men in the same boat. This is the very positive upside of Facebook.

But as true in the IVF circus as in any other area of our online, shared lives, is the fact that there's some good and not so good stuff to get involved with. And that's the point, I suppose. Walk into a newsagent and come out with the magazine you wanted, not a whole lot of other stuff. Same online. Get to hear the voices that you want and need to hear. Online is where we play out so much of our bad news, our down-on-our-lucks and our been-there-tried-that. But it's also where we share our learning, our positive experiences, our values of trust and empathy. It's a difficult balancing act: personal protection and privacy versus the opportunity for knowledge and like-minded support.

So much of research and reading around IVF is about finding out the truth. Not just the facts but the facts that are relevant to you. There's such a lot written and said on the subject, by so many different groups of people – by doctors and consultants, by journo hacks mongering the myths in the media, and by the thousands of online scribes sharing the spills and the thrills of their experiences with the likes of you and I. Somehow, you need to see the wood from the trees. It can be all too easy to get stuck or carried away with opinion forming press outings like this one – typical of its kind, and cut from any one of the last ten to fifteen years: 'The baby millionaires: Fertility experts become medical profession's highest earners. Helping desperate women to conceive earns these unorthodox specialists more money than even the best-paid plastic surgeons.'[2] Not one of the red tops, in this instance, but a Sunday broadsheet wanting to whip up a bit of moral panic, peddling the broadly held perception that IVF has an underhand side to it, run by practitioners who are getting way too rich. The article goes on to identify ARGC's Taranissi as the highest paid IVF practitioner in the UK (then). Yes, we pay people like him a lot of our money. They are highly skilled and much in demand. Fertility treatment costs a lot of money, of course it does. But like it or not, ARGC performs as ethically as any other UK clinic does, and has delivered healthy babies for many thousands of thankful women. This is the line good, high earning IVF practitioners take, justifying their work by seeing it from their patient's perspective. But it's just not as interesting a story! In searching for that balance, there's lots of good and sensitively written editorial on the subject, too.[3] You just need to find it.

Self-help – Mission in Life
One summer weekend, at the very dawning of our infertility, L and I attended a New Couples workshop, held in leafy Regents Park and run by a fabulously Californian couple, just the right side of evangelical on their subject (and book): 'The Ten New Laws of Love'.[4] Two days of these two had me in a bewildered but loved up state, dead certain that we, of all couples, could head back home,

knock out a few new laws of love, and make a decent go of our union. Suffice to say (to date!) we've stumbled through, although there's no law of love, new or old, that makes safe any of the relationship explosives laid down by infertility along the way.

The Californian couple's eighth new law of love is well worth sharing, because of the life affirming benefits it can bring, both to individual and couple, throughout any life / couple stage. Here it is: 'This law teaches that true love cannot be sustained until both parties are on some level engaged in his or her own true work. Mission in Life is partners' commitment to the fulfilment of their own and the other's life purpose. Intimates are either a mission's most powerful support or its most formidable saboteur.'

Take away the slightly New Testament tone of its voice and you have the essentials of it – some necessary life mission pursuit that is our very own, and freely endorsed by our partners. A *dream* mission, whatever it is, that isn't to do with each other, or our children, or even our calling and yearning for children. Something we want to achieve for ourselves, that is, for most of us, beyond the reach of our day-to-day lives – our work lives, homes lives, love lives. Something that promotes ourselves and is fueled by ourselves. And it's the process of that Mission, the authors pointed out, rather than the end game, which benefits and strengthens the self.

I remember L saying that she felt let down by that eighth law of new love, that her life mission *was* all about children, her own children! Nothing she felt, could replace that mission of self in her life. The one that she couldn't even get going on. Of course, she understood the theory. But the timing wasn't good, to say the least.

But it struck real chords with me, and still does. It's good to have something that takes you away from the coalface of infertility, physically and emotionally, even if it's just for a few hours, or the odd day now and again. I'm going to pick on writing – something of mine that stirs me up whenever I get around to it. Not simply because of its transporting qualities, much as I love the creative kick it gives, but because of its self-strengthening spin offs, the ways it can both reflect upon and shift how I feel about something. Intangible perhaps, but it's got something to do with squeezing out those creative processes that are juicing away inside us all.

I've always been interested in writing – poetry and prose – and most of the time lug around a notebook in my bag. For over a decade I've attended a monthly workshop, run by a writer called Myra Schneider. She's a poet mainly, but amongst the several books she has published is one called 'Writing

My Way Through Cancer'[5]. It's an emotional account, but a very practical one too, about the self-help benefits of writing through a very difficult time, like the one she found herself fighting.

She talks about how writing 'lifts her out of herself'. And by writing, Myra doesn't simply mean her poems, or her stories. She means lists, notes, scraps of feelings, events, details; a montage of what you are going through, a jigsaw of yourself, all expressed through writing it down.

Her book is an interesting mix of journal, notes, poems, and crucially, writing exercises. All of them promote the self-strengthening benefits of the process itself – getting it down on paper – rather than the finished, polished thing of a poem, or a story. She suggests helpful ways of 'letting go in lists' by writing down a whole stack of what you feel – anger, pain, loss, hope. Ways of 'visualizing' through writing what you are going through, of using writing to 'record and assimilate the experience you've been through...to explore your new perspective'.

I didn't, in any way, write myself through infertility, as Myra did her illness. But it certainly helped (and still does). Sometimes, I would find myself fictionalizing the emotional experiences of our own childlessness. In Myra's terms, 'visualizing' or 'exploring' it. A London story, for example, set three hundred years ago on the banks of the Thames (near where I live), about a market stall couple and their foundling child – a tiny baby left in a bundle by a desperate drover's daughter, along with a dozen weary geese. The couple, unable to conceive themselves, take the child in, and of course she becomes their own.

Self-help books stating the 'bleedin' obvious' (thank you, Will Self) are two a penny, I know, and this is in danger of becoming yet another on that stacked-out shelf. Self-support is a better term, perhaps. But it helps to give yourself that kind of break, keep that breathing hole clear.

Work

At one point, as one IVF cycle quite quickly followed another, L stopped working. Whilst work can be the thing that 'lifts you out of yourself', many women find only final straws at their places of work. Lack of understanding and sensitivity cause major headaches; employers and colleagues taking the struggles of a woman's treatment all too lightly, as just another of the myriad of issues they insist on bringing to work with them. I have seen it myself. Post IVF two-week bed rest is a difficult period to justify to your overstretched and cutback colleagues. But understand it they must, at least to some extent. If they don't, and it all becomes too much, then something must give. And fatigue is a real issue here. The constant self-administering of drugs and needles becomes a full-on job. We have one friend who used to make quite a show of disappearing into the ladies on a night out for a jab and a sniff. She was brave, keeping up both her workload and a full social life. But eventually it even got to her and she found herself in a necessary state of retreat.

For men going through it – in the spotlight of their own infertility, or from the shadows of their partner's – work can be a bleak, joyless place. Little place for you in the day-to-day run of the mill stuff; the banter, the jokes, the drinks after work, the usual stuff of life that gets most of us through, most of the time. Mentioned earlier, but infertility is a disempowering force, across all walks of life. And of course, apart from the obvious clinic visits, there's very little understanding for time off work. I was lucky. Much of my work throughout my time was rich and varied in people and place. My hands, at least at work, were helpfully full.

Keep busy might be a summary of all this drumming up support. Keep carefully and bravely busy. 'KBO,'[6] as Churchill used to say (although never has a mantra for life been less appropriate).

5
They're in the freezer!

After a few month's wait for her FHS levels to settle down, and having gone several rounds with Zita West's acupuncturist, L's second go at IVF was, on the face of it, a more straightforward affair. Since we had a couple of decent embryos in ARGC's freezer (cryopreserved as three-day zygotes during our first cycle), L could skip stimulation and retrieval, and proceed directly to transfer. Assuming, of course, both of them had warmed up and would grow to blastocysts, as was Mr T's plan, all in good order.

It certainly felt more straightforward, after round one. There was a minimal drug schedule, and no interference with L's natural cycle, since we weren't forcing another batch of eggs. At the same time, we wondered whether a fresh round might offer more hope. These two embryos were, after all, part of the same batch that had failed to implant less than five months previously. Nothing is overly straightforward around a cycle of IVF treatment, except the simplicity of success itself, the goal that drives us through it.

The difference between a zygote at three days and a blastocyst at five days is substantial, surprisingly so. A three-day-old embryo has typically cell-divided four/eight times (reproduced already!), whereas at five days an embryo is formed from an inner group of cells destined to become the foetus, and protected by an outer group to become the placenta, once successful implantation has taken place.

Pause for a big question here. When to put the embryos back, after three days or five? It's an issue that has attracted much debate and speculation. Lots of embryos don't make it to blastocyst stage, simply because they lack the necessary genetic instructions to go on growing (a fact that no IVF doc, however good, can do anything about). That, undoubtedly, must be an awkward explanation to give wannabe parents excitedly peering into microscopes at the wonders of their cell-dividing embryos. Hence the 'put them back on day three and see what happens' scenario. There'd be little comeback on the lab in the event of no pregnancy, since it can't be determined, for sure, whether a three-dayer was ever going to make it to a five-dayer, or whether the cause of failure lies elsewhere. You're entirely in their hands and you have to assume good clinics today are making the best judgments about implantation (when, how many and in what state), based on the available evidence they can see before them, in their petri dishes. They can't afford not to be. Certainly, as in vitro conditions and quality checks improve, then the five day put-back means the lab knows more about the potential growth factor of an embryo; about which ones stand the best fighting chance of hooking onto that lovely soft, mushy endometrium. One thing is widely agreed upon and driving the trend in their favour: that taking embryos to maximum blastocyst stage significantly reduces the risk-outcomes (to mother and child) of multiple births, since fewer embryos, typically, are transferred. [1]

I think our little treasures, fresh out of the freezer, were successfully grown into blastocyst stage, prior to transfer. What I do recall, very clearly, is a conversation with one of the lab nurses, after she had shown us our thawed-out embryos. We were asking her about her extraordinary job, its life-giving role, and of course, its flip side of disappointment. She was a friendly Australian woman, very experienced even by her late twenties, and happy to talk about her specialist subject in a confident, open manner. 'Where did she go from here?' we wondered. 'IVF consultant perhaps, here in London?' 'Nope,' she replied, her plan was to 'head back to Aus, work in the same field, but not with us humans.' 'Uh?' 'Yup, the real money,' she explained, 'was in horses.' The mind boggled for a moment. 'So hang on a minute, you're out here practising on us guys before you roll up your sleeves back home and get to work on the gee gees!' Amazing. I can see her now, working away in some Aussie equine lab, petri dish in one hand and a betting slip in the other, standing a much better chance in the Melbourne Cup than the rest of us.

Just a couple of days later, with our embryos lined up, we found ourselves back in the quiet, studious surrounds of the basement laboratory, under the spell of the nurses' hushed talk, the Starship Enterprise hum of the machines, and the steady hand of Mr T.

Bed rest, for L, wasn't too bad a sentence. She could focus on what the body was trying to do, give it the best chance of pregnancy with rest, sleep and plain, healthy food. And, as on previous and subsequent sessions, she was dealing with the energy sapping, nauseating effects of the drugs, so bed was as good a place as any to be.

Time for a few words about those drugs, and the way they affected L. Here's a brief description of what they're supposed to be doing. Common to most treatments of IVF cycles, the drugs involve three clear stages, across a long or a shorter protocol. The first is known as a down regulation of a woman's natural cycle. A drug such as Lupron for example, switches off the pituitary gland (in the brain), which under normal circumstances releases the monthly hormones (called gonadotropins) that control the action of her ovaries. Taken as a daily injection in her thigh, it suppresses ovulation, thins the lining of her womb, and induces a kind of menopausal downing of tools. Now the doctor can take control.

Once an ultrasound scan confirms ovarian shutdown, it's time for drug stage two, a synthetic version of the follicle stimulating hormone, or FSH. So a drug like Gonal F for example, stimulates the ovaries, increases follicle and egg growth, and also oestrogen (these FSH-like drugs are also used for men who have a low sperm count, due to low hormone levels). Doses are tailored to suit each woman, and are jabbed daily for 10–12 days. With another ultrasound scan, follicles are counted and their diameters measured, and the condition of the womb lining checked.

Assuming all looks encouraging, the third gear change of drug now comes into play. This is a shot of HCG (a pregnancy hormone, under natural conditions produced by the placenta), often referred to as the trigger. This pushes the eggs into a final growth spurt, and stimulates a natural surge of a hormone produced by the pituitary gland called the luteinizing hormone, (known as LH), which triggers ovulation. Egg retrieval, typically, is about two days later.

If fewer than three follicles have developed, the outcome will be poor, and usually the cycle is abandoned. If, on the other hand, a woman has produced too many follicles, she's at risk of ovarian hyperstimulation syndrome. L didn't suffer from this, but we know women who have, and it can cause severe abdominal pain, body aches and nausea. Sometimes it can be very serious.

Not surprisingly then, given the battering to her natural cycle and the stalling then rushing of her hormones, L experienced most of the symptoms as expected: extreme tiredness and loss of energy; abdominal pain (different kinds of grinds and stabs to those brought on by her endometriosis); nausea; pounding headaches and some whopping great mood swings. And I do mean whopping. Egg retrieval itself is painful, too – the follicle suction of eggs via a hollow needle probe – causing bleeding, tenderness and yes, a bit more nausea. It's a gruesome business, led by a multitude of DIY injections that none of us have any previous experience of administering.

Yes, we choose to do all this. Ultimately, L didn't *have* to go through it. Nobody does. Of course it's about choice. But equally, when life itself is clawing at you to reproduce and there are treatments out there that might stop the clawing, then you can kiss the concept of choice mostly goodbye. For many women, the idea of choice, by this stage of the game, has long since deserted them. They will take what's on offer and go the extra mile, whatever the pain.

Just as L completed her two-week bed rest, I disappeared to China for a ten-day block of work. Nice timing, I know. On the day I headed off to the airport, her first blood test revealed once again a positive result, a chemical pregnancy. Exciting news, but I knew from her voice, when I phoned her on my arrival in Beijing, that she was feeling dreadful, barely having the energy to take Jessie to the park. Jet-lagged and sleepless, I felt that I had deserted her cause, left her to her daily pregnancy hormone blood tests[2].

For a few days, six perhaps, her blood tests were encouraging. Her beta numbers were rising nicely. But then they weren't. Just like the first process, and the third a few months later, they started to fall off, and sure enough, L wasn't going to be pregnant. There followed a series of heart crunching phone calls between us down a crackling line. Phone calls made up of sobs, two-bit words of love and sorrow, and long agonizing pauses filled only with the humming silence of the distance between us.

From then on, China was a strange trip, lurching by van, train and plane from the foggy damp beauty of the central Wudang Mountains, to the big coal-mining town of Changchun in the east, near the closed borderline with North Korea. I had a lot of road-time to think. Mile after mile of suburbs and factories; huge hazy fields dotted with workers, carts and white egrets; muddy rivers full of boats; small towns of thirteen million with thousands of people meeting at dawn to exercise, or at dusk, to dance in unison for an extraordinary hour of tinny waltz. And one of the things I thought about was the one child rule. For a couple of days, we travelled with a local woman journalist. She, like the few other Chinese women we met, had just the one child, in her case a daughter. She told me about her family and after a while, I started to pry, asking her if she wanted another child. She laughed and said 'no, of course not. One is fine and allows me to work, which is what I want to do.' It was impossible to read more of her private thoughts, and of course, her mask around children seemed to mirror my own.

The last three days, as we made our slow way back to Beijing, were a miserable write off. I picked up a dose of food poisoning the effects of which

I shall never forget. I just about managed the flight back to London, then crawled into our bed, still warm from L's recent ten-day stint.

By the end of that year, we had been through three unsuccessful IVF attempts. After the third – disparagingly referred to by Taranissi as 'quite bloody' in his notes, when we read them several months later – we showed up at ARGC for our debrief. Taranissi sat us down in his office. Maybe it was a mid-afternoon dip in his famous energy levels, but it seemed to us his face was longer, and his usually bright tone of voice was dulled with one or two telling sighs. It felt like we had turned into a cul-de-sac that afternoon, as we wearily listened to what he had to say.

The gist of his prognosis was this. He suspected, though he couldn't be sure, that L's failing to get pregnant might well be because her immune system wasn't allowing her to do so. 'How so?' we asked. He explained, perking up a bit now that he could bury his long face in the explanatory folds of reproductive science, albeit an unproven and controversial one. Taranissi thought there was some credence in the idea that L's immune system was rejecting her first-stage pregnancies. Mostly, he told us, your immune system sees off invading cells that have a different genetic make-up to yours. Viruses, for example. Or a tiny embryo in her womb, that had a genetic pattern of my genes as well as hers, so is recognized as different. In normal pregnancy, it is thought the body does something to stop the foreign embryo being rejected by the immune system, though no one is sure exactly what. The immunity cells present in the blood stream are called natural killer (NK) cells, the ones that normally see off outsiders. Perhaps, the theory goes, the NK cells found either in the blood, or in the womb lining at an early pregnancy stage may be fighting off the embryo and winning out. Neither Taranissi, nor any other IVF doc, has any hard evidence around the idea that NK cells in the immune system are somehow rejecting the implantation of an embryo in some women with fertility problems. But he did subscribe to it, as many others have done. And so we listened hard, albeit with our heads down.

Mr T moved on to talk about egg quality, telling us again that never would he, nor anyone else, fully know the quality of L's dwindling egg supply. He reminded us that many embryos don't divide and grow because they are genetically impaired, right from their start. Back then, if you wanted to have your embryos chromosomally tested for their competence or abnormalities (one/six embryos is thought not to make the chromosomal grade in L's age group), then you sent them off to America. (Today, there are clinics in the UK licensed to carry out such tests[3].) He could arrange this, but he explained, with another weary shake of the head, we needed more eggs to select from than our IVF cycles were producing.

We left his room sad and deflated. Downstairs we hung around the office, L having some drugs to return. Unusually, Ellie Taranissi had enough time to stop and talk to us. The last words she said to us, as we stood amongst the nauseating wallpaper of mum and baby mug shots, were 'You'll get there. I've never seen a couple who really want a child not manage it somehow or other.' 'I have,' I thought, as we walked past that glossy gallery of baby snaps and through ARGC's doorway for the last time, out into the November damp of the street. 'I bloody well have.' Loving, strong couples that tried their hearts out for a while, but then stopped. Either they drifted apart and split up, or somehow managed to move on to the next phase of their changed lives, the one without children.

I did think, for a few days, that perhaps we'd had enough, maxed out our share of science. A friend of mine who partnered his girlfriend through several cycles of IVF calls it 'peddling hope'. I remember calling it something similar that grim afternoon, probably a little stronger. But this last attempt had left us aching for more understanding of why. If we found out why, then surely we could make it work! We knew how good Taranissi was, but looking back, I think both of us felt that something had to change if L were to attempt another cycle of treatment. A combination of Taranissi's despondency that afternoon, and his downbeat 'quite bloody' comments amongst his notes, seemed to be sending us on our way. It was time to move on. What he had done, however, was to point towards a possible area of infertility cause. And what we needed was help in trying to overcome it, some renewed and sparkier hope around sorting it out.

But first, we needed a break, a bit of mending between the two of us. Two days later, we booked ourselves into a dog friendly B&B in Sussex for a couple of nights, near Rye, and got blown away in a blast of winter sun and wind on the giant dunes and shore lines of Camber Sands. Jessie dog went joyously crazy, and the two of us dug in close against the weather, calmed by the fury of sea and sky. Except for one or two careering sand yachts, we were alone on the vast ribbed skin of low tide beach. In Rye, we had hotel tea and rummaged in a jumble sale, where I picked out a small, beautifully kept 1923 diary, written in neat pencil by a young maths teacher living in Crystal Palace and working in Sydenham. Each day records one or two gems from the achingly plain minutiae of his life: walks with his belle, Emma; Wednesday night snooker; extra maths classes for slower students; cycle rides and punctures; trips to the flicks and

Saturday afternoons watching his beloved Crystal Palace FC. To this day, it remains by my bedside, a small but totemic celebration of a year's ordinary passing in one man's life – beautifully accepting of his present, wonderfully devoid of any dreams for his future.

After several weeks of licking our wounds and trying to have a break from it all, L started to talk more with Zita West about our troubles, and about Taranissi's thoughts on NK cells. Zita was encouraging and mentioned another clinic, Sher Institute for Reproductive Medicine (SIRM)[4], based in Chicago, run by a South African Doctor called Geoffrey Sher[5]. He had, she told her, gone further down the reproductive immunology line than most, and offered both treatment and hope in overcoming it. Back then, more than ten years ago, Zita was interested in the possibility that imbalances in women's immune systems might be affecting successful implantation. Today, she continues to be open minded about the immunology factor. Whilst acknowledging the controversy that surrounds it, her own clinic takes seriously the possible role reproductive immunology (RI) issues might be playing, for a small percentage of women, particularly amongst those experiencing repeated implantation failure.[6]

When L told me about Sher, my reaction was to get busy online and ramp up our research. Spurred on by Zita's addition of a new trans-Atlantic character to our script, I remember thinking that perhaps that poor, stressed-out woman I had shared a coffee with all those months back was right, that self-gleaned knowledge was the only way forward. Empower yourself with facts and make it happen! And it wasn't long before we latched onto the line of Sher's thinking: 'More than half of women with endometriosis (regardless of its severity) have immunologic implantation dysfunction...30% of all women with endometriosis...have evidence of activated natural killer cells (NK) in their uterine linings (endometria). It is this NK activity that represents the most significant reason for immunologic implantation dysfunction in women with endometriosis.'[7]

Hard facts! At least that's how I saw them. No matter that many experts doubted, still doubt, the NK cells / implantation connection. No matter that tests and studies were, and still are, in their infancy, that not even a blood test can determine an over-abundance of NK cells in the womb lining, since they're not in the blood to test. No matter! Here, at last, was a chain of connection between L's wretched endo (as it's fondly referred to) and her failure to convince one of her embryos to take hold. At last, a line of explanation, running from Taranissi to Sher, that stacked up. (Since reproductive immunology is so often referred to across the infertility treatment landscape, and because of its controversial nature, it's worth knowing what the HFEA's position is on the subject. [8])

Furthermore, Zita told L, she knew of one other London-based woman who had pursued Sher's way and successfully produced a baby. Zita introduced her to us, and with that compelling combination of joy and success, she phone-talked L through her experience. She was, needless-to-say, a firm Sher advocate.

In terms of treatment, too, there was a hopeful way forward, something called intravenous immunoglobulin (known as IVIG, or plasma therapy). Even today, it is yet to be licensed for use in reproductive treatments, such is the lack of proof that it will increase a woman's chances of having a baby – although it does now appear on ARGC's menu (plus those of a few other clinics), sometimes with the addition of immune-suppressing steroids. But if there was truth in the NK cell immunology theory, then IVIG made sense. It is made from the antibodies extracted from the blood of many different blood donors (all of them fully screened), and then dripped into a woman's blood stream. The idea is that this somehow bamboozles her immune deficiencies – the activities of her NK cells – and so overcomes them.

So, on several peoples' recommendation, we booked a phone appointment with Doctor Geoffrey Sher, which he conducted from his Chicago clinic. Right from the start, Sher's manner and approach was big, bold and confident. He was 100% supportive of Taranissi's line of prognosis, and re-affirmed his own belief in the connections between endometriosis and reproductive immunology issues. And yes, IVIG was something he would recommend for L, both before egg retrieval and after her embryos were returned. He quizzed us about L's previous three cycles and said he would study the notes; perhaps try a shorter protocol since the longer standard one hadn't worked. It was a breezy, mostly one-way conversation, punctuated by a series of short, punchy questions, most of which L could answer. He rounded off his talk with a vote of confidence – he wasn't put off by three rounds of failure and was hopeful of success. He told us we would be most welcome at his institute and to go away and think about it.

Which is what we did, although not for long. By the time January of that new year had limped to a close, we had, at least mentally, booked our flights to the US.

6
Vegas, the final throw of the dice

It was mid-March and I had just turned forty. 'Play it quiet,' said my gut. But L sprung a wonderful surprise and flew us to Venice for a long, breathtaking weekend (can't think of a better city break from IVF, such is the gobsmacking otherness of Venice. Water not tarmac, boats not cars, for a start).

Not so wonderful was the surprise waiting for me when we arrived back home. The TV production company I had been with for a few years was having a cash flow moment and had decided to let two of us go. Redundancy. Bugger! Now I really was off the script. IVF was one thing, but not being able to pay for the bloody thing was quite another. Emasculation to the max. Losing a job is a curious thing, if it happens to you. You feel cheated somehow, sickeningly hard done by without exactly knowing why. But after a while, you also feel a brand spanking new kind of elation, as if a door has opened and you are stepping into a bright new place. That, plus a kind of healthy dose of 'fuck you'.

For L and me, it was Las Vegas that was to be the first of those brave new dawns. We had settled on the idea that our fourth round of IVF might be in Chicago, where we had spoken to Geoffrey Sher at his institute. But twice a year he took his IVF skills on the road, and worked out of a sister clinic in Vegas. And it was his Nevada clinic that he was now inviting us to attend.

Viva! Of all the places to gamble on a fourth round of IVF. Dream-fuelled Vegas, built on a wing and a prayer in a dry, stony place, slap bang in the middle of the desert. If ever our IVF lives needed a spice-up, this was our chance. From Upper Wimpole Street to Medical Mile, Sin City, the 'gambling and entertainment capital of the world'.

There were several stages we needed to go through prior to our trip, related to fertility checks or treatments. Not content with the several sperm tests I had already had, Sher wanted to check for himself the essentials of numbers and motility. No point in you guys going the distance, he suggested, if you ain't firing straight. I thought I was firing straight, I offered, but to no avail. Having read all our notes, Sher wanted to start from scratch.

Question: how to get a beaker of sperm from a rat run in West London to Sher's institute in Chicago, and keep it fresh in the process? Freeze it and fly it is the answer. Sher's people had given me careful instructions on what to do, but doing it was another thing all together, particularly with a house full of builders knocking up a kitchen extension. Time for the diary to take up the story.

28th March

Walked the dog, back by 9.15am. Eddie and the builders on their breakfast break, Eddie sitting at the table reading a biography of Alex Ferguson (it was Alex Higgins last week). Everything under control. Dry ice to freeze sperm arriving 10.00am. Courier arriving 10.30am to ship it off to Chicago. Should be fine. Thirty minutes to slip upstairs and do the necessary, seal the jar and pack it into the dry-iced container as instructed. Time to make some coffee, that's if we had a kitchen, which we don't. So I pace about, going over the plan. At least I'm not cooking all this up from work – things could be worse. There's a knock at the door. That'll be the ice, right on time. Standing there is a man in protective clothing carrying a clipboard. And beyond the hedge is his enormous container truck, hissing quietly as it blocks up the entire road. 'Not all for me, then,' I say to him, though I don't suppose he knows the purpose of his delivery. I sign, and then he pulls out a small hose and nozzle from the side of his truck and enquires where I want it. I give him my polystyrene container and feeling I owe him an explanation, tell him, 'It's medical.' He grounds the container and inserts his nozzle, telling me to 'Step back and keep out of the way.' Back at the truck he presses a few buttons. There's an intensity of hissing and then a quick release of white breath from the side of the truck when he turns it off. He advises me to pack whatever it is I need to pack outside and then leaves. Stage one, done. Right, upstairs with the plastic jar. I decide on the bathroom as my venue – I'm used to delivering in a small room, after all. Ok, here we go, nice and easy. Hell's teeth, it's the door again! The bike's early! I down tools, zip up and whizz downstairs. Opening the front door, I find not the helmeted biker I am expecting, but four men unloading stacks of breezeblocks onto our front path – from another bloody great truck. Christ, this is getting busy. 'Come on through,' I call, leaving the door wide open. Eddy ambles through the house as I take the stairs by storm. Back to it, although it's trickier to stir the senses with several beefy blokes humping breezeblocks through the house just a few feet below me. Never mind, nature takes over, bless her, and I finish the job in hand. Great! It's the door again. I tuck myself in, cap the jar and run down stairs. This time it is the biker. He waits while I nestle the sperm jar into the packaging and seal the box. I check the paperwork and the instructions. The biker looks on, a bit mystified. 'It's medical,' I find myself repeating, and shove the paperwork in the bag. And that's it, he's off to the airport and so is my sperm. Eddie shuffles along the corridor. 'Right, Charlie, we need a decision on the size of that window...'

Treatment-wise, as he had explained, Sher wanted to tackle what he thought to be L's reproductive immunology issues with IVIG, that drip-fed cocktail of other people's antibodies, gathered from their donated blood. To give her embryos the best chance of survival, he wanted this to be a two-stage offensive, at the start of her IVF cycle (now!) and then after implantation, when she was back from Vegas, during her two-week bed rest. Again, this was easier said than done, since back then, this was an unusual treatment in the UK. With some difficulty, and with the help of both Sher's London contacts and L's gynaecologist, she managed to score the necessary amount of the right kind of blood, and book herself into the London Clinic for her twelve-hour drip. The nurses were new to the protocol and it took several stabs in the back of her hand to get the flow of foreign blood flowing into her own. Once the drip had settled down, she felt no serious side effects beyond some mild headaches, and as for the nurse's blundering start, she told me it was 'no big deal,' adding that she had acquired the status of 'pin-cushion' long ago.

Sher also suspected L had a potentially embryo-killing bacterial infection called ureaplasma urealyticum, found in the cervix and vagina, and swapped back and forth between the two of us. All women experiencing infertility, recurrent miscarriages and pelvic pain, in Sher's book, should be tested for the bug. The theory – again, inconclusive – is that this infection can lead to fertility problems. Another reason, perhaps, why our previous two rounds of IVF, maybe all three of them, hadn't worked? Who knows? Certainly, it was part of the evidence bank we put together around our decision to fly to his clinic in the US. You find yourself building up a case like that, and so long as there's a strong rationale, that's OK. Proven or not, we gobbled up our antibiotics and started to think about what to pack for Vegas.

Meanwhile, L's drugs had arrived and she began her different length of protocol, as administered from afar by Sher and his staff. It was a strange time, our sense of trepidation laced with a twist of that buzz you thrive on before a trip. My current state of financial insecurity certainly added to that nervy blend – anxieties that were impossible to shelve until I could get back home and rustle up some work.

Who the hell goes to Las Vegas for just over two weeks? Our Virgin flight from Gatwick, not surprisingly, was stuffed with the usual Vegas mob: long weekend gamblers, old-timer couples wanting a bit of re-charge, gangs of families (grannies, toddlers et al), a group of girl-friends up for the party. Safe to say, no one was sharing quite the same journey as us.[1]

20th April

Leave Gatwick 11.00am and arrive Vegas 3.00pm local time. We check into 117 Homestead Suites, a spacious no-fuss room with a functional kitchenette corner, a nice big double bed, a built-in writing desk, and a small table with two chairs. As usual, I take immediate ownership of the desk (blokes!), by unpacking a few books, my computer and a pad of paper. I know I'm going to have a lot of time on my hands and plan to do some writing, at the very least make a decent attempt at a diary. L, much more usefully, takes control of the top drawer of the desk as the best place for her sizable stash of drugs. She unloads them and neatly lines them up in order. We're tired, hungry and feeling the strangeness of all this. I go out and buy Greek salad, ham & Swiss cheese sarnies at Denny's. When I return, L has put out a couple of pictures of Jess. It's the first time we have left her, and L has shifted her jet-lagged queue of anxieties onto the dog (not a bad thing, in the circumstances). She is crying. Both of us feel lonely. It is always hard telling your partner you feel lonely. The one thing your partner is supposed to be doing, simply by being with you, is relieving that loneliness. We eat and unpack. That helps. Then by 5.00pm, sleep beckons and that helps a whole lot more. Predictably, I have brought along 'Fear and Loathing in Las Vegas' – Hunter S Thompson's head bang of a trip to Vegas. I make a half-hearted start. Sleep takes over, but already it's a fast and furious read.

21st April

At 9.00am, after breakfast at Denny's, we check in at the clinic. It's a short walk from Homestead Suites. It seems we're staying on a strip known as Medical Mile, comprising hospitals and clinics, and self-accommodation like ours for people who are using them. Not the most attractive part of town, to say the least. It's warm and breezy outside, air-conditioned cool inside.

L is well into her cycle and Sher doesn't waste any time. When we meet him, he's an impressive South African/American. Like Taranissi, he has real presence. He's quite fast talking, but friendly enough. Accompanied by a small posse of nurses, he breezes into the ultrasound room, where L is already set for her first scan, propped up slightly and her feet in stirrups. He is swiftly through the introductions, and then straight down to work, assessing her womb lining for thickness, and then her follicle numbers. Like a dentist checking a row of teeth, he reads off the numbers and measurements of her follicles. She has six, maybe seven worth noting, each standing a chance of releasing a healthy, mature egg. His tone is encouraging. It's not a high score. L has had 14 before. But it's 'quality not quantity', he murmurs, more kindly gauging the four side-effect weeks of jabs, drips and drugs that L has put in, just to be here at all. Yes, we need to dig deep and be positive around the limited score, particularly with a dopey fug of jet lag still in our heads. And we know only too well that there's no IVF guru on earth who can pinpoint exactly the quality of an early stage egg. This is classified information, a reproductive secret that our biological nature, however far we probe into her, will not give up. We must sit it out for a couple of days, when egg retrieval will reveal the number and at least a shade more of their quality.

22nd April

1.00am. I awake, unsure of where I am, but now see L sitting at the desk, in lamplight, hunched in concentration over a large syringe. This is her trigger jab. It'll shock her body into ovulation and final egg growth, exactly 36 hours prior to egg retrieval. I get out of bed and pull up the second chair. I don't say anything. She's in control, although I know how nervous she is. She draws up 1cc of sterile water from one bottle and squirts it into the HCG powder in another. Now she draws up the mix into the syringe. Then she changes the drawing needle for the injecting needle, frighteningly thick and long. This one is destined for her arm, deep into her muscle. She taps out the air bubbles. On her instruction, I grip her arm, already bared, above the muscle. She steadies her right needle-hand, takes aim. She's brave alright. Not a flinch as she sinks the needle a long way in. Then slowly out, a trace of blood and a button of cotton wool over the top.

23rd April

Homestead is a bulky, bland building with thirty self-catering large rooms like ours. This fortnight, with Sher's clinic in town, it's full of IVF cyclers, although no one else is from the UK. We make friends with a NYC couple, Patricia and Jeff. She's training to be a doctor; he's a construction lawyer. This afternoon, the four of us take a drive out to the Red Rock Canyon National Park. Only a few miles out of town, it's a wild, scraggy area, loaded here and there with Joshua trees and a thick, heavily scented growth of ground level scrub. We drive all the way around the park's 12-mile loop road, stopping a few times to take pictures, walk a little, pause besides the ancient *signage of the Paiute people whose home this used to be around a thousand years ago – beautiful little handprints made in red-earth dye on the flat surfaces of rock, some kind of shrine perhaps, or notice board (another movingly kept secret). They gave us heart, these affectionate little imprints of direction, spirit and trust. And as we stood quietly in front of them, it still seemed as though they were doing something, reaching out, showing, or just about to touch.*

When we get back to town, we go for an early dinner, Lebanese. Apart from one other couple, we're the only diners. Good food, but most memorable about the evening is what happens after our plates have been swept away. Belly dancing! Here she comes, shaking her thing, making a beeline for us since there's no one else to beeline for. She circles us and then drapes her arms and hair all over us, coaxing us up to dance. Which Jeff and I do! Not Patricia and L, women in their condition. But up we get, us blokes, making some moves, plenty of hip action, hands in the air, fingers clicking. Vegas, IVF, Homestead Suites, Joshua trees, and now belly dancing with some construction lawyer I've only just met. The company and laughs does us both a lot of good, settles us well and truly in.

There's another couple we meet today, too, Lisa and Joe. Joe works for the police force in Dallas and trains police dogs. He has a beautiful large Alsatian called Dallas. We talk much about dogs, since we're both missing our hounds.

24th April

Their jobs done, at least their immediate jobs, some of the guys on the programme have slipped away, back to work, I guess. Jeff heads back to NYC, Joe to Dallas, another guy to Miami. No such easy escape for me. And it's a slightly stranger, broodier place, Homestead Suites, without the other males of the pack stalking the corridors. Some of the women here retreat further into the privacy of their rooms; others emerge to seek our company. There is, not surprisingly, a lot of chat about follicles and eggs. It's day four and we pretty much know how many vitros folks have been through, what their stories are. One woman upstairs has managed to knock out a whopping batch of 24 eggs, most of them frozen for later use.

There's maybe seven women staying here who are being treated by Sher, and today, I go shopping for four of them (including L) – food and feminine hygiene products mostly (as the marketing world calls them). I manage to limit the run to two stores, one regular supermarket and one more whole foodie store. Plenty of roughage, expensive organic ready meals, salads, cheese, comforting choco-treats. By this stage I have tamed the hire car and have got the hang of the one-way system. Everyone drives everywhere in Vegas. It's a God-given right to have a car, and everyone has one. There's more SUVs than you can count, and plenty of old road junk, too. Near Medical Mile we have a Walmart, a giant Gap, a Borders, a nice internet café, and a gym, which I have joined for the stay. Back at base, I fill the lift with home deliveries, knock on a few doors and distribute the goods. I chat for a while with Lisa, Patricia and Jade. I give them their bills, and money changes hands. Hmm. I could get used to this.

25ᵗʰ April

This morning, L had her eggs retrieved, under local anaesthetic. It's prickly painful afterwards and she feels a little woozy. No surprise that there were just the four retrieved, but the news wasn't confirmed to us without a little drama. L was lying in bed, curtained off, but effectively in a ward. I was standing at the bottom of her bed, having just been allowed in. Sher was doing the rounds with his posse. We could hear him working the row, pick out some of his hearty greetings. Now it was our turn. There was an extravagant sweep aside of the curtains. Tanned face, broad grin, one of the other nurses holding a clipboard. He greeted L warmly. 'Now then,' he said, leaning across to take the clipboard whilst ignoring what the nurse was trying to tell him. 'How have we done? Excellent work, congratulations!' This was odd. Four was fine, if the quality was up, but you wouldn't break out the fizz over four. 'Eleven we retrieved, that's excellent and now you have plenty of choice!' Oh dear. It was clear to everyone, even L through her wooziness, that he was reading the wrong line. And now he was listening to the nurse telling him so, for the third time. 'What? Let me see that,' with which he raised his glasses high on his rusty head of hair and peered at the board. 'Ah, I see, four. Well, four's OK! What we wanted! Good work, L!' And he's off – the show must go on – just time to ask how she's feeling, that she might feel a few stabs of discomfort as the local wears off. Half an hour later, we're back in Homestead Suites – via Denny's, naturally – L gearing herself up for those stabs.

At 6.00pm, L had her first shot of progesterone since her GP friend, Caroline, showed us how to do these big, intramuscular jabs a couple of weeks back. She told us that 'sometimes you hit a bone, especially if you're firing at 40 degrees to the body. If you do, you just pull out and go in somewhere else. But the needle will be blunted, so you'll feel it more as it pushes in.' Sobering stuff. Unless you're a yogic black belt, or a contortionist, large jabs in your arse are best left to someone else's steady hand. 'Shame Caroline didn't fancy a couple of weeks in Vegas,' I murmured, as I check the steadiness of mine. The needle looks impossibly large. L lies down. I kneel close and rub her bottom affectionately. 'Get on with it,' says the patient, calmly. I choose a spot, a nice chunky patch on the upper thickness of her left cheek, close to the one Caroline had picked. Here goes. Engage. The tip of the needle bites into her skin. 'It's OK, it's going in,' I mumble quietly, more for my own benefit than hers. It pushes easily through fat. Then it falters, about 3cm in. Muscle. So just as Caroline had said, I push more *forcefully and it slips in some more, until all 5cm of needle is sunk in her flesh. Now we talk each other through the next stage – withdrawing the plunger a few mm to see if there are any traces of blood, indicating that a vein has been hit. It hasn't. 'No vein? OK, then push it all the way down,' L says, quietly. So I shove the plunger down and empty the syringe of progesterone. 'All gone,' I report. Pick up cotton wool. Withdraw needle. Clamp on cotton wool. Needle safely down. Breathe. Now I peel a plaster and gently lay it over the tiny, deep wound.*

We both lie on the bed. I don't know how many more of these we're going to have to do, certainly one a day for the next eight days or so. Could be up to twelve weeks if she gets pregnant.

26th April

Saturday and we want to do something different. The wind which yesterday was gusting up to 35mph has quietened down over night and it's a beautiful spring day, temperature up to the high 70s by mid-morning. L has found a swap meet (car boot sale) to go to, so we drive out to NE Vegas and park up on the edge of the 40-acre site. Inside are several hundred cars, vans, stalls and tents, lots of people selling, thousands more drifting through the lines, looking for stuff to buy. Most people here are Latinos and a meet like this is clearly vital to their pockets (Vegas is full of work – one of the best-off towns in America – and nearly 30% of its people are baby booming Latinos, 68% of those being Mexican). L and I wander through a half mile square of the meet, whole families gathered around their cars and their wares. Pretty much everything you'd ever need is here. Old and new clothes by the ton, CDs and DVDs by the metre, lovely home stitched blankets, groceries (for people and animals), work tools by the thousands, and a choice of delicious, tangy snacks. I buy a 1958 US Army Jacket, Korea, the real thing. L says she is saving herself for Goodwill plus all the other charity stores in town. We visit two on the way home. She wasn't joking.

When we get back to Homestead, there's a message from the lab. Three of L's four mature eggs retrieved yesterday have successfully fertilized. This is great news, and picks us up hugely. L takes to her bed with a beaming smile on her face, tells me she's just about ready for the microwaved macaroni cheese I have shopped for her. There's such a long way to go – just the next couple of cell dividing days for these little fellas are major hurdles. Sher has told us he will most likely go for a three-day transfer, not five, given L's low egg count. She sleeps soundly.

I head downstairs and sit on a bench in the car park, the closest thing to a garden around here. It's a suntrap and I shut my eyes and listen to SUVs and birdsong. The wind has picked up again, and its bustle through the car park stops me from dozing off. For a while I watch it driving the spray from the water sprinklers crazy. I get out my pad and start making some notes for a poem. I try to think what it must be like, for L, to focus on the very physical sense of her journey, shape the words and the lines around the bends of its course.

Waiting for rain
In Sri Lanka we shared a stand of rain,
crowded beneath corrugated iron
with the laughing chatter of children,
the sea full of rain and all the skins of the earth
soaking it up – cattle hides, palm sides, sand,
the bare wet of their sleek arms.
Here was our first map of children,
something to steer by in the dark.
In America, thunderheads bruise the mountains.
Storm light makes immaculate angles and shadows
down the backs of the hospital buildings
where inside our first circles of life
nudge and cushion their brave beginning.
You stay in bed, drinking water
and watching the weather channel – twisters tearing
at the heartlands of Texas, Oklahoma.
You breathe in belief, let the storms chase you with them.
Sometimes it seems we have moved through these years
as if month after month were a chain of weather,
calling off searches and starting others,
or waiting for rain and knowing what joy it may bring.

27th April
The storms cause hundreds of flights to be cancelled. We watch the Weather Channel open-mouthed: shaky whirlwind clips shot by storm chasers from their car windows. Most of Nevada is safe. But the wind that brewed up yesterday in the car park is still gusting through Vegas.

We have the day to ourselves, so we head south of Vegas towards Hoover Dam on the highway. We turn off the main road and motor slowly through Boulder, the town that grew up in the 30s and 40s as a neatly laid out suburb-extension of the vast construction and accommodation camp that sprawled out around the dam.

We're parked up at the dam by 9.30am, ahead of the traffic. Hoover Dam is surely one of the seven man-made wonders of the world. It's an awesome place, powering and *watering most of thirsty Vegas, much of LA and other vast swathes of the West. Every inch of this dam, interior and exterior, is beautifully designed, its great curving flanks plunging down to the Colorado River, way, way below. It has all the breathtaking scale and detail of the Chrysler Building or the Empire State Building – from the heroic, pencil shaving smoothness of its sides, to the Olympian elegance of its detail, every brass railing, elevator button and brushed steel finish.*

The building of the dam attracted attention across the dust bowl of work-starved Middle America like nothing else of its time. At the feverish height of its construction, in the mid-to-late 1930s, around 3,000 men showed up for work at the dam, thousands more loitering around the peripheries of its site. Most of them went hungry and lived with their bedraggled families in a vast makeshift slum known as Ragtown, sprawling for miles beside the river. For the lucky ones, life got better and several hundred of their families were even housed by the company. But the work for most was dangerous and hard. Amongst the toughest jobs was that of high-scaling – guys dangling on ropes down 1000ft of hard rock face, drilling holes to shove explosives into. Once they'd lit the fuse, they would dance across the cliff-face to the relative safety of a flimsy wooden perch, stick their fingers in their ears, and start praying. For this, they received the princely sum of $1 per hour, twice as much as the rest of the crew. Nobody got buried alive, the guide merrily told us, and only 95 men died on the job. L said she could barely look at the photo-portraits of the Ragtown men, women and their scrawny, serious-faced children.

We stop at Lake Mead, the largest man-made lake in the world. We pay $5 and drive down to one of its beaches, a muddy half-mile foreshore. I go for a swim. It's still chilly from the snowmelt Colorado. Out of the water it's hot and burning, so we don't stay for long. Oddly, there's a swarm of large ladybirds. They bite the crap out of me whilst I'm drying off.

28th *April*

Transfer day. We hang around our room most of the morning, not wanting to miss the call from SIRM giving us an update on how the three chosen embryos are doing, and what time that afternoon Sher wants to put them back. Around midday, it comes through. Of the four that were retrieved, two have cell divided well (ten and nine cells respectively) and one not so well, just five, although apparently it might catch up in the next few hours.

Another small victory. Our margins for success weren't terrific from the outset – six follicles, four eggs, three of those successfully fertilized, now two, maybe three good to go back to their willing host.

We have two hours to kill, so we drive a few miles out of town to see the acupuncturist recommended by SIRM. This will calm L's nerves, settle her uterine cavity (how these terms are tripping off the tongue these days!). I sit with my notes on a scrap of turf in the sun. Her place is on the edge of some characterless shopping mall. Two rednecks climb into their truck, fire it up, screech backwards and then wheel-burn out of the lot. Christ, I could do with a few of those needles myself.

Last night we turned the Weather Channel off and had sex. Probably the most unlikely sex we have ever had, certainly amongst the strangest. Sher asks all his IVFers to have sex the night before transfer. Why? Well, he has a hunch that it helps – something in the fluids that is good for the transfer environment, beds it all in. Another bloody hunch. I wanted to hold back, perversely, to not come inside L, even though (for once) coming pronto was what we were after. L thought I was overcomplicating the matter. So I came quickly and thought about the environment. Then we kissed and went to sleep.

L pays her acupuncturist who says she'll see us later, post transfer. I'd say L is as calm as she'll ever be, given the circumstances. We head for Homestead to pack a day bag. It's time to see how steady Sher's hand is.

Once she is horizontal and waiting for transfer, L isn't allowed to pee. Her full bladder enables Sher's ultrasound scan to read the uterus cavity more efficiently. Poor her. She's bursting for an hour while she waits. At last, she's wheeled into position. Another curtain is whipped open and Sher strides in, flanked by his trusty embryologists. He doesn't waste any time. First he lets a bit of L's pee go via a tube (painful). Next he's calling for the cathode tube, inside of which are the embryos in their uterus-like liquid. Now for some more, good news. The little guy embryo number three has caught up, just like they said he might, and is now a healthy enough, cell-divided seven. All three are going back. Sher is upbeat, positive, delighted. Then hush descends. He inserts the tube and glances at the screen. He's already done a test measurement of her uterus cavity. Now he releases them, by sight, working through her distended uterus opening, and happy with their mid-uterine position. He quietly talks us through his progress. There's not much to see on the screen, just a disturbance in its middle. And now, for a moment or two, he does nothing, remains still, transfixed. Then he eases out the catheter and hands it to Dr Levant, the embryologist. Levant scurries off to check whether all the embryos have been transferred. Yes, they have. L is tilted back on her bed, legs pushed together, and then lowered. She's told to stay calm and still for an hour. Sher is pleased with his work. He turns to me and shakes my hand, twice. Then he clutches L's and tells us there is 'nothing more I can do. Now it's with the hands of the hands.' And then he leaves. I know there's a tear in my eye, so there must be several in L's.

Dr Levant is in his late 30s and has a calm, intelligent way about him. He returns from the adjoining lab room to give us a full embryo report. I like this level of dialogue between us, something we didn't get in London. SIRM have their own method of scoring embryos to rate their transfer potential, based on rate of cell division over three or five days, depending on transfer day. Anything above 70% he explains, is rated good. We have two over 80%, but the catch-up guy, at 65%, is an outside bet. He tells us he's been with SIRM most of his embryologist life and we get the feeling he's one of the inner-circle few round here. He's wonderfully positive about our chances, and tells us he believes wholeheartedly in the potential of our embryos. He shakes both of us by the hand, then leaves.

L is pushed (nicely) aside into another curtained-off room where the acupuncturist's needles are waiting for her. On her second strike of the day, she must think it's Christmas. I can't help thinking L is surely getting enough bloody needle action without this lot. But that's between me and the diary.

We arrive back at Homestead just in time for L's backside shot of progesterone. Since the last one, we've asked one of the nurses to re-show us the juiciest jab zones, and just for good measure, circle them with her pen. Now I have something to aim at. L also starts her twice-daily jabs of heparin again, thinning the blood with the aim of further tempering her immune system.

Then she takes to her bed, where barring trips to the bathroom, the drugs drawer and one or two gentle journeys out, she'll stay until we leave town, in six days' time. On her bedside table is a black and white printout of her three cell-divided embryos – perfect spawn-like circles, one of them with its cells already merging together. Even with this smudged little picture, it's easy to imagine their tiny fizzing pulses of progress, already forcing themselves at the boundaries of their beginning.

1st May

L is set up with her book, drinks and meals. I take off for the day. I drive back to Red Rock Canyon, this time paying to enter the conservation area within the looped drive we did the other day. I have picked a walk I want to do, a seven-mile circuit around the wide base of White Rock Mountain, called White Rock/La Madre Spring Loop.

It's hot, around 30 degrees, and the air drying out as the day warms up. After an hour or so, I'm at the westerly elbow-point of the loop – furthest away from the road and Vegas beyond. I'm still in the looming hush of the White Rock's shadow, have another hour to walk in the shade of its hood. I pause and face west, the mountain behind me. In front of me is a vast wilderness of scrub-sided scraggy slopes. There is no wind to speak of, just the faintest push of air now and again, but I can hear the great howl of its silence, the slow, hollow moan of the ancient, dry-bedded canyon. Somewhere behind me, up on the side of the mountain, rocks fall. I turn at their cracking and scattering of dust. Nothing there to cause their falling. Not a soul to mark the passing of canyon time. I think of the small, tough, Paiute people that lived here a thousand years ago. How they found and touched each other's lives, how they somehow managed to give birth, feed and raise their young.

I think of L back in our Homestead Suite. As I see her now, she is neither asleep nor reading, but holding the scan of her embryos, fixed on their shape and form, willing them further into the thickness and safety of her womb.

Out here, in Vegas – the place to which we have travelled so far, in pursuit of so much – L is very focussed and emotionally quite calm. Everything else is on hold. It helps, in a way, to be so far from home on this leg of our journey, to grip the process of IVF so differently. I let the rush of the canyon's great emptiness mass around me. If I get lost out here, if I stumble about for days, then I will begin to feel as she might have felt, some of these last several years. She's right. Nothing else matters, at least not for now, not until we're through with it all.

An hour later, I stop for water and listen for tortoises. It seems like a good place, lots of low scrub cover and small ledges of rock. The book says sometimes you can hear them before you see them. Desert Turtles, they call them in Nevada. I wait to see one's scuffing paddle through the stones. Eventually there's a tiny kerfuffle, but no turtle. It's a lizard, a perky little lizard.

About halfway around the loop, I watch the high thermal turns of an eagle. It mews a faint, high rasp of a cry, kitten-like with distance.

Near the end, I begin to see a few other walkers. It's cooler, and there's a mile of track, closest to the car park, where dog walking is allowed. Vegas folks love their dogs. These are the heartier types, yomping the trail in their sneakers, their hounds – ridgebacks and labs – loping along behind them. Back in town there's a magazine called 'Vegas Dog'. L loves it. There's a particularly camp section on day care for dogs. The more you pay, the more your pooch gets pampered. $60 a day buys your little yapper the full hotel experience – doggie TV, bed service, endless grooming and cuddles. Only in Vegas.

Back at the car, I drink water and rest before driving home. I feel full of heat, my trainers and socks red with trail dust. My heart pumps away. I feel thirsty but sated and stirred by the canyon's might. There is nothing I can take back of my walk for L, save this, my descriptions. But I have broken from our routine and now I am ready to return to its main event.

2nd May

Joe, the policeman from Dallas is back in town, to re-join his bed-resting wife. He invites me out gambling. L says go, she'd be with me if she could. Chucking money at the tables with a Texas copper! The script thickens. Joe's no stranger to the scene and shows me the ropes. We agree on $80 each as a sensible figure to lose, $100 tops.

We go to Caesar's Palace, one of the older casinos tacked onto the vast hotel of the same name. Around the casino is a kind of mall, full of food and drink joints, frat bars most of them, judging by the clientele. Fortunately, we've chosen a place full of Americans not Brits, at least not the shower we flew out with. The casino glows a kind of a crushed red, the kind of light you want down there, I suppose. Beers and some of the spirits are free if you're playing. Girls drift around with drink trays making sure no one is empty handed. The whole place is a tightly run ship. You get the feeling a lot of staff are tucked away watching surveillance screens. Roulette – holding your breath for a land on red or black – doesn't do it for me. But the craps tables are fun and neither of us (quite) loses our limits.

Joe's a friendly, calm guy. We steer clear of IVF chitchat and when we're not talking about how to win money, we talk dogs, which he knows a lot about. He's interested in Jess and gives me a few tips on training. Like J is for us, their dog is their missing link of a child. We head home around 2 in the morning, early for a tinsel town night out, back to the much more important dice we've been rolling along Medical Mile.

3rd May

L feeling strong and bold. We go out and eat at a great little Mexican café, wedged between two quickie marriage chapels. Afterwards we drive to the Elvis Museum, and then the Liberace Museum. L adores both and scores a fine selection of cards and fridge magnets – Liberace (avec his fluffed-up pooch on top of his piano) in full make up and glittering jewellery being the favourite (rumour has it that he made his partner have plastic surgery so that he looked more like him!).

On the way home, we park up across the road from the iconic 'Welcome to Las Vegas' sign. There's no high rise here, just the faded, original 50s style motels and storefronts. We cross a lane of cars and take each other's picture beneath the candy-pop sign, even find someone to get a shot of us both. We've arrived! Vegas has us strangely under its spell. L takes it gently, but for a few releasing hours, our time here feels more like everyone else's. We're on the trail, taking the same famous pictures as millions before us.

5th May

I take the hire car back to its base. It's time to say goodbye to Vegas. Unlike crazy man Hunter, who smashed his car through the perimeter fence, we take the more usual route to the airport, in a cab. Yesterday, we said goodbye to Dr Sher, his right-hand woman Linda, and his chief embryologist Levine. They have one more two-week cycle *to perform before they pack up shop and head back to Chicago. We've become friendly with the whole crew. They've looked after us well, and there are hugs, kisses and handshakes all round.*

Sher's post-transfer words are rattling around my head: 'Now it's with the hands of the hands.'

7
Turbulence

The flight home was, without doubt, the worst I have ever taken. L kept her cool, remarkably, and just as well given the valuable cargo she was carrying, but I certainly didn't. The journey started well enough. I had booked us economy tickets, but a friendly woman on the Virgin desk fixed us a pass to the lounge, so we could administer the jabs in relative comfort and privacy. This we did. They even let us stay there reading and snacking until the flight was called. But as soon as we were herded into the economy cabin, which was packed out with returning holidaymakers and gamblers, I had a strong sense of what we were in for. Three hours into the eight-hour flight, turbulence struck. Amongst tipping trays, stumbling aircrew and cries of passenger fright, L's shut-eyed face went pale, her gripping knuckles white. When she could, she had tried leaning her seat back as far as it would go, only to be met with repeated back-of-the-seat thumps from the moronic (hung-over) guy behind her. I asked him to stop, added the word please. He asked me what my fucking problem was. I didn't have the bollocks to tell him exactly what my problem was, and anyway, accepting his invitation to step outside wouldn't have been an option, even if I had fancied my chances. So L and I changed seats. I was furious, with myself mostly, for not having predicted this cursed leg of the journey home, and for not having bought her the upgraded comfort she should have had.

Several bouts of altitude plunging turbulence later, the worst either of us had ever experienced, I vowed to remove L from her economy seat and into a more horizontal position. Once I was free to move, I went in search of the most senior crew member I could find – the red-suited woman from upstairs in the first-class bubble. I told her our story of the implanting embryos. Pleaded with her to let L lie down somewhere, whatever it cost. She told me there wasn't any room elsewhere, no spare seats in business or first. What about crew beds? Or premium economy? All of it met with more shakings of her head. I told her about the scary guy behind us. That didn't work either. I did the pleading all over again, more desperate this time, and produced SIRM's notes on jabs and bed rest. All to no avail. I asked to see the person in charge of the flight. She was in charge, she said, apart from the pilot and his chaps up front. Could I see the pilot, then? Nope. So I let her have it. I told her she was being unhelpful, unsympathetic and not acting at all in the way you'd imagine she might if you believed all that Virgin PR shite. And just to finish up, I asked her under what circumstances would she ever consider helping a passenger? If they were actually *having* a baby?

Flushed from my rant, I returned to my seat. I wanted to bury my head and cry, or hit someone, preferably the bloke behind us. Neither of which would have got us any closer to getting the baby's bonnet made. L told me to calm down, she was OK, and that there was turbulence in business and first class, too. We held hands for much of the remaining trip, and eventually, got through it.

Home was a strange place to settle into, when we got back there. After the comparative safe haven of our Homestead Suite, and then the trauma of the flight, it took most of the remaining days of L's bed rest for us to re-gear for home, to be in charge I suppose, now that we were off Medical Mile and a long way from the clinic. I think we felt exposed, prematurely let go. And, of course, we had left Vegas and its veils of real and unreal behind us. People run away to Vegas, to get married, lost, laid or loaded. And most of what happens to them in Vegas stays in Vegas. They leave it there, sheepishly returning to the more regular run of their lives. But not us. Just like other folks, we'd gone there to find what we hadn't been able to find anywhere else. But unlike them, we'd brought it home, the dream held tightly between us.

However, the daily business of L's jabs steered our days, those big progesterone suckers in her backside (the biro targets, I made sure, were still there to aim at), and we were doing everything as per our instructions.

L re-housed her treasured embryo printout beside our bed, and spent her time reading or sleeping or pottering about our new kitchen extension (the one Eddie the builder was working on when the dry ice arrived). There were a few finishing-touch decisions still to be made – floors, tiles and colours – just the right amount of distraction from the nail biting wait for her tests (the quantitative beta HCG blood pregnancy tests described earlier). She also had to get her row of ducks lined up for the next few weeks, her final session of IVIG at the London Clinic in Devonshire Place and the venue for her blood tests in Harley Street.

She spoke with Zita West, always calm and supportive, and the nice woman who had successfully undertaken the US/UK Sher process was willing to be on the end of a help-line. As with previous legs of our journey, what counted was the endorsement and encouragement for what we were doing, and the more personal the connection along the chosen route, the better.

The weather was very hot those early May days, touching 90 degrees in London (98 if you happened to be sitting on the tarmac at Heathrow Airport). Jessie and I went out running or walking in the early mornings, sticking to the shady-green tunnels of the riverside path. Then I painted the back of the house, and when I'd finished that I set about re-laying the lawn. All decent distractions, not least from the fact that I was jobless and we were at the end of our financial tether.

I was fretful this time around, a bit fearful, despite being the seasoned IVF campaigner that I was. And my feelings were stirred by concerns about money: I was now face to face with the employment coalface from which I had recently been laid off. The work ethic runs so deep and strong and this – a first for me – was a time when I had nothing in the pipeline. But I think, too, that I was fearful of what was next, of the script drying up if L's result went the same way as the previous three. And whether, in the face of repeated failures, it was going to be possible for us to re-write it at all. There was perhaps, an inkling from us both – unspoken at this stage – that our IVF reserves beyond our current efforts were beginning to run low.

But we got the house and garden straight and soon enough, test day came around. This time I went in with L and waited while she went into the lab. More than five microliters of HCG per ml of blood tested would indicate that her embryo(s) had implanted. Or at least had tried to. That's the science. The reality is much, much more gripping.

I sat in the waiting room, or rather paced up and down its confines. I thought about going outside to walk the street, but I didn't want L to return to an empty room. I was nervous. I hadn't forgiven myself for the plane ride home, and now the terrible episode was running riot in my head. Surely all that bloody turbulence and thumping of seats had taken its toll?

Twenty long minutes later, L re-joined me. She had a beaming smile on her face. A result? Yes! As we headed for the car, she was quick to point out that a second test was needed for confirmation, but for now, she was quietly glowing with pride and pleasure. When we got home, we rang up SIRM and told them. They were delighted too, albeit cautiously so.

For nearly three weeks, the rest of May, her tests remained positive, the numbers doubling up, more or less, pretty much as they should. And just for a moment, the odd hour in amongst these treasured days, L allowed herself the unadulterated pleasure of being pregnant; of actually *feeling* pregnant. Nobody was bouncing from the ceiling, and hardly anyone knew of her progress. Of course, it was way, way too early for that. But for her to feel, just for once on this tormenting, bloody ride, that she had earned her place, her goddamn rightful place! Christ, what a warm, momentary joy for her to savour. She'd ring me up and tell me how she was feeling as she made her way home from the clinic, freshly laden with news of her rising numbers. And once or twice, when I returned home after a walk or a Sainsbury's run, I'd find her pottering about the house, the rest of her life contentedly and wholesomely lost within this new and glowing sense of herself.

What ever happened, L told herself, then she had owned this much, felt and known all that this meant. The call of her nature was being answered as never before (the one that tugs at the sleeve of all our natures at some point or other, the one that never really gives up, no matter what you tell it, or where you put it). Somehow she knew she had to bottle it up, keep this quiet acknowledgement and achievement close, know that it was properly there for more than a blink of an eye or a beat of a heart. Physically, she began to feel different, too. A slight soreness in her breasts. One or two symptoms, however small, of early pregnancy. And so we began to believe, and this time we had something more to pin it on.

At crunch times in our lives, we're prone to lean a little heavier on our gods. I am not a churchgoer; a respecter of other people's gods without being a believer myself. L, though, was raised a Catholic, a Spanish Catholic at that. And when she feels the need for a quiet word with Himself, she heads up the road to St Mary's. Once a Catholic always a Catholic. Now was certainly one of those times. Off she went to commune with her God, thank him, assure him that she would do her bit, keep her side of the bargain. I think for her it offered a channelling of hope, a different kind of time when she could filter her yearning for a child through the spiritual and cultural process she was brought up with. A few minutes when she could make a quiet bow to a benign force she felt to be far greater than herself and her own limitations. But it worried me that she might see our lack of conception as a failing, in a Catholic sense, in the eyes of her God; as if somehow there was something to forgive, which he must've known there wasn't!

A few words about God and infertility, whilst we're on the subject. Several times I bumped into Himself when talking to people about IVF. A conversation with strongly Catholic friends of ours about our infertility treatment never got off the ground, certainly not into the realms of the rational, and in the end, we agreed to leave it. And on two or three occasions, people I talked infertility and IVF with delivered that knock out line that goes something like, 'Well it wasn't meant to be...' And spoke it with that kind of god-spooky shine in their eyes. They meant it! Really did think that something else may be at work here, other than the two of us and the glorious randomness knocking around our lives. A god who not only chooses who has children but also by which method! I admit to finding all of that very hard to take. I know they meant well. But I found it just about the most unhelpful thing anyone ever said to us around our infertility. And that includes some real quacks and hacks we met along the way.

At the beginning of the third week, on her fourth or fifth test, she was given a due date. That's right – given an actual due date. I have often wondered why. Protocol, I suppose. Some doc or nurse just doing their job, naming the day. L knows that January due date as if it were tattooed on her arm. I don't. But this wasn't meant for me, this strange date lancing off into the future. It was hers, her very own. A date she will harbour for the rest of her life. And looking back, although it worried me at the time, I think that nurse did the right thing, however unwittingly, however premature the date for the diary. She was helping L build her case, adding to the tool kit something else to feel pregnant with, to touch the beginnings of that special state that so many women get to feel – lay their hands on their tummies and know that their lives will never be the same again.

Well, I guess you can sense where this is going. Just a day or so later, L felt a change. A physical change. Nothing big to begin with. But something she describes as a kind of leaving. And sure enough, by her next test, the progress of her pregnancy had slowed. She began to know that something was up. You never fully know why, or how, at this awkward, too early stage. But if the numbers aren't rising sufficiently, and consistently, then the prognosis isn't good. Somehow, the implantation is failing. For the unluckier few, it can be a first sign of ectopic, or tubal pregnancy. But she felt it losing its grip – her tiny, embedded embryo. Felt it letting go.

Two days later, May Bank Holiday, L felt a series of abdominal pains: pulsing, regular throbs. Spots of blood soon followed. She phoned her gynaecologist and talked through her symptoms. Already aware of her recent run of results, he wanted to see her as soon as possible and booked her in that afternoon at the Portland Hospital. Again, we found ourselves in a hospital waiting room.

But this time, we knew what was happening and what the result would be.

The Portland was Bank Holiday quiet. Very few staff, no other patients milling about. Presumably women were delivering away upstairs, but we didn't see any of them, nor any of their blanketed little bundles on their way out to a waiting car. We met our man in Reception. He greeted L kindly and took her off to a treatment room. I remember, whilst sitting in the hum of the waiting room, focussing intently on the fact that we had been allowed to park our car bang outside the front doors of the Portland. How fortunate we were, I kept telling myself, to be able to park right outside, what a difference it made! Odd, the small, simple brain tools we use to get us through such difficult times. And I remember thinking L was being treated by a caring professional she would trust with her life, that if anyone was going to deliver the final blow, then he was the man.

There was, of course, nothing else for me to do, except keep myself sane over the next half hour or so. I was shocked that our Vegas IVF had come to this. It didn't seem real that it was over. But it was, and in the fish tank quiet of the hospital, the state we were in began to hit home. Like most men would, I put my head in my hands and let my clenched eyes squeeze out some of their tears.

Her gynaecologist examined her carefully, his ultrasound scans finally revealing her empty egg sacs. Sure enough, she'd had a very early miscarriage. Back in Reception, he told me how sorry he was. Then he turned to L and said a heartfelt goodbye. It was time to go. We sat down and let him leave first. At this point, L had a license to collapse. But she didn't. The reserves of resilience, calm and pride she had treasured and saved these past few weeks now came into their own. She was, even now and despite her condition, starting to move forward, beginning to shift this loss and all its preceding losses, into the rest of her life.

In time, I began to see that she had loved these past few weeks of bat-squeak pregnancy more than anything else in her life, more than me, more than her family, and in a sense, more than her own life itself. I was deeply moved by what she showed me of herself that strange afternoon. And I was immensely proud of her, too. It was her that led us out of the hospital and back to the car, her that put a best foot forward.

8
When enough is enough

It was time to drag out the script. The bloody thing needed re-writing. But not quite yet. L needed a rest, a change of scene, a change of personnel. We both did, before we could decide what was next.

Describing an IVF attempt as a cycle is biologically accurate. But I had begun to see it as something else, more as a 'bout'. Something with a bit more body blow to it. Four rounds with IVF had left L bruised and jabbed, inside and out. Yes, infertility treatment had given her a choice; empowered her. And this can't be overestimated. The UK average success rate is creeping up (now over 20%). It can and does work, up to 40% of the time! Brings babies to couples who couldn't otherwise have their own; a gift of science – so long as there's a realistic chance of success and everybody knows the facts – that is hard to argue with. But there is a cost, a mental and physical cost that won't be ignored.

IVF has been around a while, fifty years or so, but still not enough time to measure the long-term effects, if there are any, of the drugs. We simply don't know, and as ever, research throws up a variety of views. One will tell you about an increased chance of ovarian cancer, amongst those who have undergone IVF. Another will tell you that there is no evidence to link the two. Remember the arguments raging back in the 80s and 90s about the side effects of the contraceptive pill? One Sunday supplement would expose a threat, only to be slammed down by another a few weeks later. Led by media outrage over its costs and its practitioners' earnings, we're not far off that stage in the theatre of IVF, although of course the pill involves many more women.

We know one or two women who have battled bravely through seven, eight or nine attempts, women who have stopped only when they have succeeded in having a child. Every woman, every couple, I suppose, has their threshold. L and I both knew, although a realization not fully fledged, that most likely, our time with IVF was through. For a few months, we battened down the hatches and tried to return to our other, more normal lives. We had been through a huge emotional and physical process, shared its short-lived triumphs and its letdowns. It had led us by the nose, this hybrid animal of gut desire and assisted science. Now it needed to be led out to grass.

Within a few weeks of L's miscarriage, we spoke to Dr Sher in Chicago. He and his right-hand woman, Linda, expressed their genuine concern and sorrow for us. Sher's opinion was that L's window was closing and closing fast. If we were to go again, he said, we needed to move fast. But the issue of egg quality was uppermost in his mind, and most of our conversation that evening was about donor egg. We agreed to think it all over. (Note to self: must get that bloody window fixed!)

For many women in L's circumstances, this would have been the next logical step. Skip the egg quality issue and go with a donor's egg, as best matched as possible. If we were to consider it, we thought, then let's stay in Europe, save our air miles for pleasure. A few weeks after speaking to Sher, we got as far as having one brief conversation with a clinic in Italy. There, as in many other donor countries a couple can have more choice and agency input when it comes to donor matching. In Italy or Spain, women are decently paid[1] to undergo the complex process of donating. So it follows that there are more eggs and their donors to choose from.

But for L, this was a period of IVF closure, not a change of its course. I don't think it was about hitting any walls, or panic buttons. It wasn't as dramatic as that. She had, quite simply, arrived at the finishing line of science and its treatment as a way through. Another couple might have pushed on. But we were sensing, more and more strongly, that enough was enough.

Around this time, we also discussed and researched surrogacy. We were introduced to a woman who had two children, both carried by a surrogate. She was happy to talk on the phone. But it wasn't a lengthy call, and afterwards, we found our feelings around surrogacy led by its issues and potential upsets. In the UK, there are no legal binds around surrogacy.[2] This was a worry that we couldn't see beyond. It didn't feel like a route for us.

Quite quickly, surprisingly so in a way, we stopped considering donor egg as an option. Or any other assisted reproductive route, for that matter. It's curious, what works for some people, and not for others. We know a couple who have two terrific children, both of whom were donor egg assisted, as today a growing number[3] are. For them, it had seemed the right thing to do, the next, most natural leg of their journey. Ours, eventually, would lead us through a different pass.

When the break came, for L, it came once again in the shape of America. Just a few months after her final round of IVF, she found herself saying yes to a work trip, yes to a stint in New York City.

Having spent most of her working life in TV production, her last three years of freelance work – when she had felt strong enough to tackle it – had been with post production companies (editing, special effects and computer animation), the last of which was called Smoke and Mirrors. They were firmly established in London, and with the market quite buoyant, had decided to follow the lead of one or two other London companies and take a pioneer leap across the pond. As one of the resident producers in London, L's turn to nurture the fledgling New York office had come around. She jumped at the chance, saying yes pretty much straight away. It was December, and anyone who has been to NYC around Christmas time will know what a special place it can be. There followed, over the next eight months or so, a valuable series of three-week stints in shimmering New York City.

London was infertility, IVF, disappointment, a city full of mothers and buggies. London was grief, and month after month the haunting, bloody reminder of her failure to conceive. It was the city of herself, and everything it had boiled down to. And London was me, too, the man she was vowed to, for better or for worse, but the man she couldn't give to, share with, have that thing with. Of course, L couldn't have said it quite like this (perhaps didn't feel it quite like this), so I'll say it for her. It was time to change her hand. Time to chuck us all in. That first trip, that pre-Christmas bolt up the arm that was NYC, was a beautifully wrapped gift of perfect timing. It was just what she wanted, and even more importantly, what she needed.

When I asked her the other day what was the most freeing thing about that time, she replied, without much pause, it was that nobody knew her. Nobody knew her via her lack of children, her agenda of infertility, her IVF, her time on the goddamn baby clock, or her bed rest time off work. She wasn't being defined by all that. She must've told one or two folks, but most of them were meeting her just as they would meet any other woman: someone good, helpful and fun at work, someone to meet for coffee and flea markets, cocktails and dinner. In NYC, she could switch to glorious radio silence on the baby front, tune in to different New World channels. Most tellingly, I think, she has never found so much simple pleasure in her own company as she did in New York, before or since. Every walk out with herself was a tingling pleasure to her being, every Bowery or Brooklyn or East Side amble an absolute joy. The gridded map she followed hundreds of times became the chart of her new life, and all its streets, work places, shops, people, cafes and bars, powerfully felt as the greener shoots of herself. It was cold in NYC that first Christmas trip, snow swirling down as she walked through its drifts in the streets. L hates the cold. But she made a glorious exception that winter.

Over the next several months and trips of a few weeks each, I made one visit out to see her (any more than that would have felt like an invasion!). She was staying in the iconic Beekman Tower, East Midtown, just south of the hulking Queensboro Bridge. In three days, we walked miles, stayed out late, partied, went to galleries, still found time for an hour or two in bed. It was one of the outstanding times in our lives together, like we were dating again. And for L, this whole period was like that, although the most meaningful person she was dating was herself. It was wonderful to see her on her new patch, so invigorated, so free from the last few years.

And, of course, it wasn't so easy adjusting to the weeks at home in-between her trips. Jess and I met a tired woman at Heathrow airport, just before Christmas after that first trip. It was tough being back in London, back in the old base. One three-week trip was nowhere near enough. I knew she needed more, and whilst I inevitably felt let down by her absence now and again, I could see the benefits of what she was doing, for both of us.

It was a regenerative time for me, too. This was the break we needed from each other's lives. I was landing some work, including another China project, and it was a relief dealing with the logistical challenges of filming in China knowing L was nurturing her self-esteem in America, not being hit by the tail end of a failing cycle of IVF. And when I was back home and not working, I'd walk miles up the Thames towpaths with Jess, spend hours pottering contentedly about at home. Our feverish concerns, anxieties and responsibilities around infertility, for each other and ourselves, had flooded our lives. Compassion fatigue if you wanted a diagnostic term for it. Now we were letting some of it go.

One of her breaks back in London coincided with her 40th birthday. Oddly, we share a birthday, March 13th. So we decided on a joint party, albeit a year on for me. It was a fabulous evening and L looked stunning. Most of the people she wanted around her were there (and a few from NYC that weren't), some of whom she had struggled to engage with in recent years over motherhood and children. But as with New York, this wasn't about any of that. Not once, to my knowledge, was it mentioned, by anyone. It was about friends, our family and us. L rode the wave of her 40th birthday beautifully that night, and through all the dancing, drink and laughter, gave all those fruitless years a right royal send off, showed them the magisterial middle digit.

Looking back, I see now how fortuitous this time apart was. Without its adventurous kicks of new and different, and despite our very purposeful goal of a child, that sense of previously identified drift in our shared lives may have taken more of a hold. It's bewildering how close a relationship can seem, even in its raw emotional state, and yet still be on the drift. There's a sense of passing each other, of losing those handholds, and in the big-time tragedy of failed life plans – the baby script – it is all too easy to give in to the perverse mind cravings that tug you away from the work of your relationship; to greener grass, somewhere else to deal with the drift on your own. And they are perverse, these demons that riddle our lives with our loved ones. Because route one, so obviously, is to get through the difficult times together! Yes, we had the infertility project together, and were tackling it as best we could. But the project had become the main job of our lives together, leaving the weekend time of our marriage fallen by the wayside. And it's a bugger, because you can't avoid it, not altogether. You need to tackle infertility with such all-consuming, intensity of purpose. The very same intensity, tragically, that catches you broadside and sets you inevitably adrift. There's the rub. And once you clock this, then you've found a further wedge-driving sense of helplessness that works its way between you. It's not as if someone else has nipped in and nicked it, the precious core of that life together. No one else was involved. But at the same time, at the base of it all, it *wasn't* our faults!

So here was the gift of our chance to rake in the rewards of time spent apart. A break from the day job, the freedom of a dozen weekends on our own. You have to get hold of the drift together, somehow, before it puts too much water between you.

The woman who returned from America, about ten months after her first trip, was healthier, stronger and despite some NYC withdrawal symptoms, more confident in every way. Inevitably, her homecoming meant something of a return to her struggle with infertility, to the inside workings of that same old couple trying to find a way through it. All the issues were still there, all the bear traps. But we'd turned a corner and were ready to get a hold of that script.

9
Adoption,
the long way home

On long walks with Jess, we would tentatively map out what was next. Not surprisingly, the idea of adoption was beginning to loom large in our thoughts.

In some ways, this next period, eighteen months or so, was one where we felt most clarity around our infertility and what to do about it. We'd closed out on the IVF phase of our lives and felt ready to get back in the saddle, albeit on the back of a different horse. Quite soon after L returned from the US, the thought that we could wrap our lives around an adopted child began to feel not just real, but the right, breakthrough thing to do.

So often when you read or talk about adoption, one of the first things that always crops up is its slowness, how long it all takes. It's curious what a bad press our adoption process gets. Insensitive social workers, care homes stuffed with hard to place kids, desperate couples held in line. These are the stories that make the pot-boiling cut. And that's a shame. However slow the process can become, however stuck in the waiting room you might feel (again), there are plenty of well matched, well facilitated adoptions going on, achieved in difficult circumstances and resulting in some terrific family lives.

The current government, just like the last several, is endeavouring to increase the number of children adopted each year in the UK. To at least shift the perception around adoption, so that it seems easier, and less slow. One of the ways they might do this is to change adoption-matching protocol around ethnicity. For many years, the prevailing wisdom in the UK has been same, same: children fare better if they can strengthen their own identity and esteem through matching the ethnicity of their adopted parents. And this makes sense. But it's a framework that can naturally slow a child's chances of placement, whilst they wait for the right match of parents to come along. Not surprisingly, they often don't, and the child remains in care (we do know of one Anglo-Lithuanian woman, living in Hammersmith, who lo and behold was perfectly matched).

The US takes the opposite view, actively encouraging inter-ethnicity in adoption. Anything's possible in amongst the American dream and its people, whatever the evidence screaming otherwise from the streets. A little naïve, the UK thinks. Probably somewhere down the middle lies the best thinking. But certainly, the speed of adoption process is faster in the US than here, and so proportionately, there are many more placements state by state across America. (What I don't know, again proportionately, is the comparative success and failure rates of those speedier and more ethnically-mixed placements. Here in the UK, you rarely hear of a placement that doesn't result in a permanent home for a child.)

Simply put, the sad UK fact is that there are far more children needing to be adopted than there are prospective parents for them to be placed with. Furthermore, most children placed for adoption are toddlers, between the ages of one and three years, rather than younger babies. Few babies are adopted at younger than six months – by UK adoption law – and in most recent years, fewer than 100 babies under the age of twelve months have been placed. The older the child then, the harder it is for the adoption team to find an adoptive home. Tragic but true.

All of this means that the backlog of children in care, waiting to be permanently homed has been steadily growing, peaking at 93,000 in recent years. In 2013, only 4,724 children were adopted from care. By March 2015, the figure had increased to an encouraging 5,360. Some proof perhaps, that government and local initiatives are finally beginning to hit home, although latest 2017 figures[1] are back down to 2013 levels.

As many good stories as there are amongst those new permanent families, and as fantastic a job as those foster parents are doing with children still in care, it's a state of play that makes you want to weep. No wonder successive governments want to speed it all up, create swifter more flexible frameworks, and more effectively grab the attention of us good folks who can't make their biological own.

A main reason adoptive parents wish to aim for young toddlers is because of the widely shared thinking that attachment and bonding might be harder to achieve, for both child and parents, in the case of an older child. A child of six or seven may have already experienced three or four foster care scenarios and so take longer to believe and trust in the permanence of their latest home (although attachment and bonding time varies and is an on-going process). A different kind of care and attention to adoption issues might come into play with an older child. Tough stories of a four or five-year-old taking a couple of years to feel at home are not unusual. The truth is that most prospective adopters have their hearts set on as young a child as the current system and their circumstances can provide them with. They may have given up on the biological route to a baby, but not the baby aspect itself.

L and I weren't about to buck the trend. The slings and arrows of infertility had drilled us very, very hard down this line. A babe in arms is what we were after, no doubt about it, not a more senior toddler. I don't know anyone who has been through IVF who sees it any other way. Yes, we knew the heartbreak facts around older children. But that wasn't a route for us. Ours was a script that still had a baby in it.

It was this that drew us strongly towards intercountry adoption; one in particular, our old friend the US. In most states across America a pregnant woman, once she has decided to place her child for adoption, chooses her child's prospective adopters, with the help of her chosen adoption agency. And once her child is born, she has three days, by law, in which to change her mind and raise the child herself. (About one in four birth mothers in the state of Texas, for example, make a perfectly understandable U-turn. Tough on the prospective adopters, but that's the idea, after all.) Six months in the UK before a placement can take place, three days in the US. That's quite a difference in adoption law, and one that struck us powerfully.

There was one other reason why the US was turning our heads, L's especially – her Spanish roots. The idea of a Latino American baby filled the Spanish part of her heart with joy. And given what she'd been through, that was enough to give mine a shot, too.

In reality, UK practice around ethnicity matching does not apply to UK couples that are adopting from overseas – obviously so, if you think of the numbers (for example) of Chinese children that have been placed with UK adopters (until quite recently, when placements from China have slowed almost to a halt). That's because international law comes into play, US adoption law in our case. The UK recognises US adoption law, so gives way to its thinking – that placing a Latino or African American child with Caucasian adoptive parents is OK, even though it (currently) doesn't agree with it. It's always struck me as a strange anomaly this one, one scenario for domestic adopters and a very different one, if you choose to pursue it, for intercountry adopters. But there it stands.

With 18 months behind us since our final round of IVF, L and I declared our adoption plans to our local borough, Hounslow, and by Christmas of that year had completed a compulsory two-day intercountry adoption course. Then in January we commenced our home study, planned for most Saturday mornings over the next ten weeks. Things were beginning to move quite quickly and we were fully absorbed in the process. We were both feeling a whole blast of fresh air.

Talking to people outside the adoption loop about all that we had to go through – weeks of social worker home-study visits with that hefty Form F3[2], being cleared by panel, then by the Department of Families, Children and Schools (DFCS) to adopt from abroad (and that's before any matching work starts!) – the response, not surprisingly, was usually one of shock horror. 'But you'd be great parents! Christ, how much proof do they need after all you've been through!' That's all true. Going through all this, you might feel exposed and tested in ways that other prospective parents aren't. But I never saw it that way. Perhaps by then we were used to putting ourselves through the wringer, or got lucky with our home-study process. Our assigned social worker – chosen for her experiences in assessing potential intercountry adopters – was thorough and rigorous in her work, but she also brought a warmth and charm to our Saturday mornings, and we grew to like her very much. Having not had infertility counselling of any kind, I mostly found both the self and couple analysis supportive, although we didn't talk to her in quite the raw way you might to a counsellor. And unlike a counselling session, where often there's an intentional and explorative sense of not quite knowing where you're going, these mornings took a very structured and focused route (they need to, there's a lot of ground to cover). The three of us were working towards a clear goal, to sail through the adoption panel thumbs up, come the appointed day. But having to write and talk about ourselves – our strengths and weaknesses together and apart – threw mostly restorative light on the difficult journey we'd been on. Most of all it did give us a much fuller idea of what we might encounter down the adoption road.

Whilst busily engaged with writing our home study tome, I had plenty of time to consider fatherhood. In fact, you get several intensive months to work on the kind of mum and dad you think you want to be. A course in parenting that other folks don't have to take. On paper, I was becoming a most outstanding dad, and L a blindingly talented mum.

Before planning to be a dad became a full-time job, fatherhood, as it is for most men I guess, was a cumbersome idea, one that lumbered along in the background of my life. You spend most of your younger adult years avoiding it, until that is, it's suddenly upon you, in all its glory. Hopefully you're ready for it when it comes along; that's about all you can hope. But infertility had me prematurely unpacking the parent within me, awkwardly picking over its bones well before the appointed time. And it was the same for L. Several times we'd both had our expectations and timings on parenthood roughed up and raked over in a series of shock waves and false dawns. I must say this did shift during our run up to adoption, changed for the better. Perhaps it was the end-of-the-road factor, or the framework and third party support that the home study schedule provided. For all its process, there felt less of an assault on the sensitive business of wanting to be a parent, and not being able to make it happen.

I know there are lots of men who don't feel comfortable around the idea of fatherhood through adoption. I've met several of them. You get that slight sideways look, the faintest not-for-me shake of the head. The thought of loving and raising a child that isn't biologically theirs is a challenge too far. And I can see why, particularly when most men don't have to think any further on the matter. Like father, like son. A chip off the old block. This is heavily encoded man-stuff, buried deep within our gender and culture. But by now, I wasn't feeling any of this. The shock of discovering that my son or daughter wasn't going to happen in the usual way was a long way behind me. So were a lot of plastic beakers and cliff-hanger days waiting for science to help us over the line. All that had long got rid of any distant, fatherhood idea of what felt natural, or mine. And when you get to the stage of considering donor egg as a route to a baby, you're a long way out from biological base camp. Certainly, the leap from donor egg to adoption never felt that huge.

There was one aspect of prospective parenting, however, that I did find difficult to deal with, harder than L I think. Every adoptive couple wants to adopt a healthy baby. But you have to consider the realities of what an infant might have been through, both in utero and during their short life prior to being placed with you. Sooner or later – about two thirds of the way into the home study (they warm up to this bit) – you encounter a thorny question: what kind of disability or birth issues would you be prepared to deal with? We knew we weren't cut out to care for a child with a long-term physical or mental disability. So we wrote that down. But the rest needed much more heart searching, reading about and coming to terms with. This bit is tough.

At the very least, a birth mother and father's medical, social and personal histories might have several chapters missing (sometimes there's nothing at all on the birth father). OK, you understand and accept that. Obviously, you get to see the hospital birth records and this tells you a lot (placement being as it is in the US, very close to birth), through the screening that has taken place – HIV, Hep B and C, for starters. But what about degrees of alcohol and drug dependency? A child whose conception was the result of rape? Or one born with a disfigurement (treatable, perhaps), a serious cleft palate, for example? And what about a child who has a chance of developing a life-threatening condition later in life? What risks do you feel comfortable with? Comfortable! Christ, what a moral minefield you have gingerly stepped into.

Drug use, for example, throws up a whole catalogue of issues, whether that use is prescribed, social (in America, it is estimated only 20% of women who smoke give up their smoking habit when pregnant!) or illicit. Some substances cross the placenta more harmfully than others, causing less, more or sometimes no damage depending on *when* during the pregnancy they are taken (a foetus is particularly vulnerable during the 3rd and 8th week, less so before). There are many worst-case scenarios. Opiates – heroin, methadone, morphine – cut mercilessly across the placenta with (often undersized) babies suffering withdrawal symptoms just a few hours into their lives. Alcohol carries all the attendant risks we know about, foetal alcohol syndrome and its grim symptoms being the worst of them. This is scary stuff to consider. You're not just reading about it in the abstract; this is stuff you might bump into, for real. And because you very often don't have the full set of facts laid out on the table, you can't possibly foresee all the birth realities that might hit home. Yes, you can decide what you don't feel up to caring through, and declare your boundaries fair and square, but you have to accept the possibility of something unexpected cropping up. There's a variation on all this for intercountry adopters who are being placed in countries like Russia, for example, where they may have to face the facts around the health and condition of an orphanage child they have come so far to see. Or, of course, for domestic adopters, coming to terms with any possible issues that a child in care might have.

But the American one that rattled me most was crystal meth. It's a relatively young and highly addictive substance, chemically concocted from over-the-counter prescription drugs. A full picture of its effects on pregnancy and infants is only just taking shape, but like the rest of the A list, it has substantial impact on growth and development of the foetus, and on the undersized baby, once it is struggling with its own dependency. I found myself gathering all my adoption anxieties around a very worst-case scenario – Middle America, its rural heartland of white trailer trash revved up on crystal meth, us ending up with a dopey baby we couldn't handle. Bloody hell! Yes, an irrational fear, since it was only one of many adoption scenarios, all of which we had final 'yes' or 'no' over should they come our way. But this was the one that went bump in my night and kept me awake. Shameful really, to let a fit of the moral panics get me like that, to feel those kinds of personal prejudices well up and muddy the whole point of adoption. But I don't suppose I was alone as a prospective adopter in bringing that less savoury part of one's self to the table. It was something that needed to work itself out.

Spurred on by our social worker, what eased all this was some of the right kind of reading. True to form, L read most of the books on the reading list and I read some of them. Two or three stood out, but none more so than the first I read, a modestly slim book first published in 1989 called 'Adoption without Fear' by a well-known US adoption worker called Jim Gritter[3]. This is a guy who helped pioneer open adoption, a new perspective that turned adoption practice in the US profoundly on its head. Outspoken, terrier-like in his beliefs and marked by his refusal to be sugar-coated, he shows through case studies how open adoption aligns adoptive parents, birthparents and child (appropriately) in a parallel cause of extended family, replacing the bygone culture of secrets and lies (as well-intentioned as they may have been) with truthfulness, cooperation and respect. The birth family are elevated within the adoption triad when previously they were marginalized, and it is the adoptive parents that necessarily facilitate this. Simply put, everybody works to put the child's life values and truth story first. It commences with birthmother choice over whom she'd prefer as adoptive parents, and progresses through degrees of openness from there. In the best of his case studies, everybody benefits. Jim explains: 'I think important ground is gained when the issue is framed in terms of the child's interests and needs. Lots of handwringing is set aside when we recognize that the adoptive person is entitled to her birth family. He or she has done nothing that ought to cost them the satisfaction of knowing their first family.'

Jim's book (he's that kind of author – you feel entitled to call him Jim by the time you're through) well and truly turned our heads. Now fully endorsed in the US, more and more openness, in broad terms, is being embraced here in the UK, too. One more quote from Mr Gritter, perhaps his best known, 'We should not be asking who this child belongs to, but who belongs to this child'. Once we were thinking like this, we knew we were ready to join that long line of people before us who had made or extended their families like this. Adoption was feeling *natural* and something people had been doing for thousands of years. Surely we could make it work!

Joyously for them, I think our families began to feel the same way. One Saturday morning, my mother told me, she had suddenly seen a bit of light. She was doing the Waitrose run and waiting in line to pay. The woman at the counter started to talk about grandchildren. Mum switched to default mode, as she had got so used to doing down the past few years. Let it pass. The buggers will talk about something else in a minute. But then, she said, she had a blast of positive feeling that it would happen; that we would adopt a baby, and that yes, she would have that grandchild that everyone asked about, have that picture in her bag to show when anyone asked her. A small but significant moment.

Not long after we had been cleared by the Hounslow panel, and were twiddling our thumbs waiting for the DFCS certificate of eligibility to intercountry adopt, we made contact with a UK support group, all of whom had adopted from America. We spoke with a dear man called David about the experience he and his wife had of adopting their son from Portland in the US. It was a great story, the first like this we had heard, first hand, and both of us were shivering with excitement when we came off the phone. David and his wife generously invited us to the group's mid-summer gathering, and there we met adopted children of all ages, their mums and dads, and one or two couples just like us, who were waiting in line. It was a magical day. That evening the weather was humid and buggy, but our mood was anything but. The light was brightening at the end of the tunnel.

When the call came, it was just as shocking as the folks in Jim's book had said it would be. It was a Tuesday evening and I was driving home, listening to the radio and thinking how the early September light was already losing its grip. Rory, from our agency in Austin, announced herself in her long, slow-bouncing, Texas drawl. She said if I was driving, then maybe I'd like to pull over. I was, so I did, illegally. She said maybe I needed to take a deep breath, so I did, legally. 'OK,' she said, 'here goes.' She told me there was a baby boy, just six days old, healthy and doing fine with a foster mother. Our file had come up, and the birth mother, with the agency's guidance, had said yes. Pause. Fuck me!

Cars streamed past. I could see the river's oily bulk glistening in the fading light. Never before, at least never quite like this, had my life seemed so burstingly sprung open. For a moment her voice drifted away from me and became a series of frayed, lulled beats, my only sense being the pulse of my being bubbling away inside me, a kind of junior chemistry set of garden shed experiments all fizzing off at once. If this were a scene from a movie and I were the guy you'd been rooting for, then this was the time you'd be stiff with fear that I might blow my chance – because instead of shouting 'Yes, yes!' and seizing it, I'd zoned out, run outside to shout at the moon, or gone into town to celebrate.

When I tuned back in, I told her I would call her back in an hour or so. She said 'Sure' but we needed to work fast. She could give us three days, tops, to make up our minds. She'd send us through all the information she had – birth family profile, hospital records – and ask the foster mum to email us some photos. Then it was down to us. Rory closed out her call. 'OK, Charlie, good luck, y'all.' I was more illegally parked than I had realized – a slim piece of red-route verge between the south bank of the river and New Covent Garden Market. But I put the hazard lights on and phoned L.

Sometimes our partners, for all their worth, are as weak and needy and indecisive as ourselves, just when we need them least to be. And sometimes they're beautifully strong, commanding and knowing. L was firmly in the latter camp that evening. All that night, she was calm, serenely sure of all that was happening so fast. By nine we'd already spoken with the foster mother, and we'd printed out a picture of the tiny smidge, a fluffy lamb tucked into his side. 'There he is,' L said, quietly and steadily, as we looked long and hard into his sweet, screwed up little face.

Come Saturday morning, just four days after that first call, we were on a BA flight (enough of Virgin!) to Dallas and then onto Austin, to link up with our agency and meet the boy himself. L had chucked in her job and I had nabbed some paternity leave (from the same company that had made me redundant two years earlier). Armed with a new camera and a book called 'What To Expect', we spent most of the flight – when we weren't pinching ourselves or easing our way with a gin and tonic (some flights are made for those, and this was one of them) – trying to settle on a name. Like any prospective mum, L had been keeping a list for years, bravely chalking up names against the run of play. Now it was time, quite suddenly, to pick one of them.

All these years in the waiting room and we still weren't ready! No name, no baby room lovingly DIYed back home. Just a few things in the hold beneath us – a Moses basket, one of those lovely soft, waffle-like baby-blue blankets, a pair of mouse-sized socks, a few other treasured things that L had dared store away in her bottom drawer down the years. Of course we weren't ready, despite all those raw parent-itching years. Being ready is a risk you can't take.

It was midnight by the time we'd wrangled the hire of our car, been to 7-Eleven for some basic stores and checked into our family room, home for the next few weeks. It was still steamy-warm outside in the car park. That day the temperature had touched 102 and tomorrow was forecast for 104. We slept sparsely through what was left of the night, our jetlag stirred up by a potent mix of anxiety and edgy excitement.

Early in the morning, before we got dressed and drove out to the agency, we lay in our bed and got close and warm against the drone and chill of the air-conditioned room. We kissed and started to make love, in that sleepy, strange-room kind of a way. But then we stopped and stayed still, ceased to continue this life-itself event, both of us finding ourselves utterly overwhelmed by what was about to happen. For a strange spell of time it was uncontrollable, monumental: fear and thrill knotted up between us, the storm of the moment clocked in each other's eyes. A son. An adopted son. Suddenly our personal narratives collided with those of the baby we were just about to meet and slammed into the here and now. Us, our families, our lives, our infertility. Him, his birth family, his infancy and the great plane of his future before us. Christmas! How life-changing can a morning be? We got up, boiled a pan of water and made tea. Then we prepared ourselves as best we possibly could to go out there and meet our boy.

Forty minutes later, around 9am, we parked up outside the adoption agency. Before we reached it, the door opened and there stood Sandie, the agency foster mum, beaming into the heat, a blanketed bundle of tiny baby in her arms. Within seconds, she'd greeted us and handed her bundle to L. We both peered in. Large, bug-eyes in his little pug face peered back; shocks of black hair; several burbling bubbles popping from between his lips. L was transfixed, speechless. But I heard her thinking, quietly and calmly to herself: there he is.

Two hours later, just twelve hours after we'd landed, we were back at the hotel – our *family* room – with a tiny baby. He was just eleven days old, barely six pounds in weight. But we did what any new parents would have done, rolled up our sleeves and stumbled into it. For a couple of days, hardly daring to believe, we shut the door and buried ourselves in the profound discovery of our different lives. There was no one else but the three of us. No family pouring in and out, no friends and flowers, no new dad (me!) getting dragged off to wet the baby's head. Just the extraordinary headlong rush of it all – lullaby-hushed sometimes, a right old mother hen of a flap other times. Hours would pass, night or day, both of us drenched in his being there and his needs – his sleeping, his breathing, his grackles and gurgles, his bottles, nappies and baths. And his crying, of course. If he wasn't in his basket, or kicking on the bed, the little guy was draped over L's shoulder or snuggled into her arms (I got the odd look in too). There she was, settling contentedly into the fog of new motherhood.

By day three the temperature in Austin had cranked up to 106. I started to venture out. We needed baby milk, nappies and stores for ourselves. It was way too hot to be out. Most folks slid themselves from their air con cars to their air con work then back to their air con houses. Outside was for idiots and losers. And bonkers new dads from London. Being a walker, I walked to the shops. When you walk the streets in any other US city than NYC or perhaps San Fran, you get plenty of 'you crazy fucking guy!' looks. The only other people out were hobos and drinkers, drifting slowly down the streets, holing up in doorway shade. They left me alone, too slowed down to care.

Come day four or five we began to drive a little further afield, early morning or evening, when the heat was off the boil. A trip to the paediatrician, meals out, visits to see Leanna, his delightful and very experienced foster mum with whom he had spent days three to nine of his life, now only too happy (much to our relief) to take us under her wing. And for me, a stack of nervy and daunting paper work – his passport and visa – sorted out from a desk lent to me by the agency.

Out of all the snaps we took during those first couple of weeks in Texas, there's one or two that will always pull the strings. One of them features the Post Office, in downtown Austin. We were fixing the baby's passport documents prior to issue and they needed to see him and his papers in the flesh. At the time, Austin was packed out with storm migrants – thousands of folks having driven in from the Galveston Gulf Coast area to escape the swirling eye of Hurricane Rita (there was one family of five camped in the hotel corridor outside our room). The Post Office had drafted in scores of staff to deal with the onslaught of communication needs, and it was several of these people we found ourselves telling our story to as we waited in line – Latinos, mostly, or African Americans. And when I asked them if they minded having their picture taken with L and her baby bundle, four of them downed tools and willingly joined in. Dressed in their light blue shirts and grouped around L in front of the mailboxes, it's a picture that speaks of everything and everybody that was good about that cross-pollinated American leg of our journey, their faces (smiling, proud, gentle or tough) a chorus of life story, tolerance and possibility. For a moment, they'd stepped away from the pressures of their own lives to share in this time of ours. It filled me with hope and gratitude that morning, and it still does now, several years later.

Rita eventually hit land on the 25th September, just a few days before we flew home. It spared Galveston, but the fourth-most intense Atlantic hurricane on record ripped through southeastern Texas, a few hours' drive from us, causing $12 billion worth of damage as she went.

When the time came, his passport and visa safely secured, we packed up our family room and drove northwest to Dallas, where we stayed the night with friends. Next day, we flew home – a dreamy, turbulence-free flight, very different to our last American exit, from Vegas. One more photo shared: L is sitting in the plane, just before take-off, clutching her bundle of beady-eyed baby. For a moment, she has turned her eyes from his to look across at me. She is smiling and her face is streaming with tears. She still can't believe it. We're on the plane, flying home, with a baby.

Our storm chasing was over, at least for the time being.

10
The afterwards of infertility

It took a while to get used to the seismic changes within our lives. Like it does any new parents. Our stop-start journey through infertility had been overtaken by that of our baby's new and demanding life. God knows we'd got lucky. A door had opened, we'd crashed through it and now we had our son. But for anyone who's been on the journey, and whatever the outcome – babies or not – infertility and its echoing experience of loss doesn't go away, at least not entirely. It goes on writing itself out, playing its shifting roles down the years.

Many times, I have thought about my friend's loss of their baby the same day as it was born. I mention this again to keep some perspective on this entrenched sense of loss we felt around the child we so badly wanted but couldn't have. Of course, it wasn't the same as that sudden brutal shock experienced by them. After all, nobody died in our story. And yet, and yet – having felt the accumulation of its absence over the years, its whacking great no show in the core of our lives – it *is* akin to the grief we experience when somebody we're close to is no longer with us. It is, in its coded ways, its own brand of grief.

If grieving around death is dealing with the loss of someone we love, then grieving around infertility is dealing with the loss of someone we crave to love. The child you will never see, never hold, love or eventually let go. And if grieving is about the loss we feel when a tightly held bond is broken, then infertility is that in spades. That's what we feel – men and women for whom the most natural thing on the planet doesn't happen. Women (even) more than men – the bonds between their selves and their fertility, their cycles, their eggs, their embryos, their hearts and minds...Those are the very real bonds that are broken. And it must be taken on, this grieving that comes our way. The less you look it in the eye, the more it'll get to you.

The trouble is there is nothing tangible to hang it on, nothing to focus it on. There's no ceremony to gather around, no funeral, no memorial service, no finally putting it to bed. That's why friends, perhaps, find it so difficult to lock onto. They can't see the way in, because there are none of the usual signposts, none of the usual props to rally around. It's an alien, Neverland place. A woman can't weep and wail at work, can't explain to her boss – not fully. None of it's like that. She can't even take a few weeks' compassionate leave (not without her colleagues thinking she's gone nuts). And even if she could, there's nothing actually there, or happened, for her to do anything about.

One of things counselling professionals seem to agree on is that you should try to grieve out each of your infertility stages, before you take the next step (certainly our local adoption team wanted to see that we had achieved this, when we eventually shifted our infertility focus from IVF to adoption). Each failed cycle of treatment, for example, every cast-aside egg, every false dawn down the adoption road, or the eventual decision to go the distance without. Get over it before you tackle what's next. Whether you can or not, when it comes to it, is another matter. Can one finger and feel grief quite like this? Repeatedly work those five textbook stages – denial, anger, bargaining, depression and acceptance? Yes, time always helps, to some degree. But I never saw L, or anyone else in the same boat, rustle up an ordered, tool-kit response to her loss quite like this. No, what happens is jerkier than this. One morning you wake up and feel sufficiently OK about it all to have another go, strong enough (just) to be waved forward by those life-craving forces, even if your heart still hangs from your sleeve. And as a man in this precarious balancing act of a partnership, you just need to grit your teeth and hope you have the strength to react as best you can to your partner's new-found resolve.

Intense, prolonged grief is hard to bear and hard to live alongside. I know this not because we weathered its extremes ourselves – not the level of sustained, permeated depression I'm talking about – but because I know couples who have, decent people who couldn't bear the pain of having it between them anymore. So, they split up – pretty much the only option left open to them – and take their pain with them amongst the rest of their baggage. Every couple wrestling through infertility has had a sniff of this, an acrid sense of where the rifts and the drifts and all the miscommunications might take them. If one of you gets stuck beyond retrieve – or seems that way to a weary partner – then no amount of compassion, support or plain old marriage vows can be relied upon to see you through. Lots of couples split through infertility, and not always at its most obvious stage of attack. That sense of loss and its effects on ourselves and our partners can go on leaking its occasional slow drip for many years, even during the successes of achieving a family (yup, even when you've got there!).

Several years away from the front line of IVF, we don't experience our infertility as those monthly thumps of loss anymore, nor the de-railing thing it once was. It doesn't eat us up like it used to. The pavements and coffee shops are no longer *only* full of baby buggies and their smug pushers (Christ, it was a shock when I realized I was now amongst their ranks the first time I shoved the buggy up the high street!). And of course, we have our son. Our son! 'Isn't that enough? Doesn't he fill that bloody absence?' I hear you ask. How could he not! His boundless energy, his twelve-hour perkiness, his laughter, his falsetto banter, that heart-gripping ability to be so willingly, so lovingly *our* son, always so firmly in the present. No, the absence is not about him. He's a key player in the script, carrying an irreplaceably large chunk of the story. But the afterwards of infertility is ours. It's about us, not him.

Here's one way it has cast its shadow over our more recent lives. Within a year of adopting our son, we started to talk about adopting again. It's a shock to any man to see his partner disappear into the fog of new motherhood, and all that it brings. Sure, you get used to it, before you settle into the idea of getting around to another. But the strange two-legged marathon we'd just completed made me cautious, and caution soon gave way to concern that another whole phase would risk the safe-haven of achievement we had just attained. I just wasn't ready to wind it all up again. But L was keener than I was, and she still is to a diminishing degree, to this day. And now I think I see why, at least in part. Her yearning for, and anxiety around, not having a second child – for our son's sake and for hers – is something to do with that deep-rooted panic response to her infertility and all the loss it entailed. But now it was surfacing through a different blowhole: she was summoning up the original loss of her biological child and gathering it around the potential loss and the very real absence of a second adopted child. More not happening. Projection, I think it's called, in counselling speak, probably of a negative variety. Of course, there were good reasons for us to adopt again. Everyone with one child thinks long and hard before they pull up the drawbridge on the idea of a second. This is natural family building stuff. But infertility meant the whole second child agenda became a more loaded issue than it otherwise might have been.

Absence of a second child. I now see that secondary infertility[1] (SI) and the kind of grief that comes with it, can be locked into any of the ways a second child might be longingly tried for – biological, adoption, whichever. (SI doesn't make room in its definitions for a second adoption scenario: it clearly needs to). The absence is deeply felt, even if the first child came as naturally as falling off a log. It's a surprisingly common and little talked about phenomenon.[2]

For the record, we did try to adopt again, from America, but it didn't work out. A combination of complications and the non-sync phases of our own stalling saw us retreat from the front. Since then, we have thought about starting it up again, domestically perhaps. Now in my 50s, it's my turn for that rattling old window to be closing. L's is more bravely ajar. So on we go, seeing every so often that ghost of infertility past. Maybe, as the years slip by, it's not even about the second child any more, but simply the tamed, nagging version of the demon itself. Just the fading clank of those opening/closing windows. And perhaps that dimming sense of absence we now feel is the acceptance stage of our grief, our infertility seeking out its final resting place. It's hard to pin down, but it's there.

Before the agency in Texas started to match us, they had us over for a compulsory two-day adoption training course. Running the session was an adoption social worker called Janie. She was funny, smart, warm and uncompromising. She meant business but she went about it with a brilliant lightness of touch. On the second day, having skilfully gathered a general feel for the personal journeys in the room, she spent quite some time talking about this baby grief, and all the loss it means – for our relationships and for ourselves. She stressed how real it was, how differently people experience it, and the kind of issues it might bring up, now and in the future. Then she wound up the session by sharing with us several quotes, from men and women living with infertility. There were some very moving lines. But the one I shall always remember was this one, written by a woman who had known her infertility for many years: 'My infertility resides in my heart as an old friend. I do not hear from it for weeks at a time. And then, in a moment, a thought, a baby announcement or some such thing, and I will feel the tug. Sadness and a few tears. And I think – there it is, there's my old friend. It will always be a part of me.'

I love this quote – the American way of it, the straight shooting, every day, little bit cheesy, openhearted reveal of it. Here's a woman's voice that drills into the gutsy core of our shared experience, the long-suffering heart of it. Who knows whether she wound up with a child or not? It doesn't matter. Her words throw light on the afterwards of our process; not just hers, but all of our works in progress. And when I think of those words, I can imagine her life moving forwards, that sense of unfinished never far behind her, but quietly unknotting itself as she goes. And I can see the shadow of her old friend waiting in the wings, the same old friend as ours, waiting for another tug at her sleeve.

11
Other voices

Today, if I look at infertility forums and groups, there is a scattering of men talking about their issues and experiences, many more than when I was in the thick of our treatment. It's great to see a Facebook group of men sharing their thoughts and support, their victories and losses, and of course, their anger at what they and their partners are going through. And there are other books by men out there too. The pack ice is being broken up, and not just around infertility. Awareness campaigns about prostate cancer for example, telling us men it's time to talk. ARGC, the London clinic we were attached to, provides a link to a large, well-managed forum called Fertility Friends[1], complete with a men's room section. All good. But then I see it's the only section of the forum – across an active range of sixty or so subjects – to have an exclamation mark announcing its presence. And the pub-like subtitle, a place for the lads to chat! As if somehow, we need all this jollity to get us stoked up and talking. In addition, several of the chat lines are started by women, the unwillingness of their partners to participate palpably clear. More women use online forums and social platforms than men. Fact. But perhaps it's time to lose the shock horror! bloke talking! factor. That might get a few more of us in.

Certainly, there isn't anything approaching a kind of collective voice yet, around men and their commonly held experiences of infertility.

Think of the volume of shared voice, amongst women, around pregnancy for example, or breast cancer, or increasingly infertility. It's a real *place*, commonly and beneficially felt by entire sections of society. Now see the gap between that, and what men don't have, around such an issue. There's the real measure; a huge amount of ground to make up.

To contribute to that slow build, and returning to the sense of shared journey referred to in the opening page of this account, here are some other personal stories about infertility, from men I have met along the way. I am very grateful to them for sharing them here.

Matt

I have worked really hard to earn the title: International wanker. Back when I was fifteen, never did I imagine – when I was locking the bathroom door for some private me time – that I would become a semi-professional at this.

Soon after I met my wife Tara, I took her for supper and she told me her ovaries twitched when she saw babies. Weirdly I thought this was the best thing I had ever heard and we got married pretty quick – both of us excited to start our family.

The challenges of infertility followed soon afterwards. Over the next several years they gained in severity and pain, at their worst when we watched a lovely friend who had agreed to be our surrogate give birth to our dead baby at twenty weeks.

After the first few months of marital bliss and no pregnancy we didn't feel too concerned. But after a year of seeing everyone else get pregnant straight away, we knew we needed to seek out some help.

Eight years later – after thirteen embryo transfers, two surrogates, one termination (chromosomal problems), seven miscarriages, a final egg donor and a trip to Utah to watch our daughter enter the world – we now have two children.

When we got married we were young and naive like most newly-weds, entering our union of thick and thin, sickness and health. But you don't really, truly understand the meaning of those words until you are faced with the challenges.

The process was so intensely difficult and draining, and as a man it is gut-wrenching to watch your loved-one struggle and not become the mother she so desperately wants to become. It goes against all your primal instincts to fix things, to look after and protect. Every friend who announced a pregnancy would leave Tara feeling teary and sad. I felt helpless and wounded every time. All our fertility problems were down to Tara and her body. She worried enormously about it being her fault. I tried so hard to make her feel safe, to know that we were in this together and that it was definitely our problem.

Another huge strain are the finances. Such a heavy load on top of the emotional one. Again, the urge to provide and look after is there and the pressure of all your dreams lie on this huge gamble of science and finance. And so totally out of your control.

On top of having to see Tara's pain was the feeling of being suddenly catapulted outside of the camp – the one full of friends becoming dads. A silent anger and a deep sadness grew where previously there was none. Smiling on the outside but actually resenting those mates and their chats about baby gadgets and Bugaboos.

Throughout everything, I feel Tara and I have managed to remain friends. A strong team. We dealt with all the traumas and disappointments with a level of humour (often dark!) that we're fortunate to share. But we are not the same people we were. And we are not the same parents we would have been. Holding our two children a little too tight. But we are through it, and it was most definitely worth every minute of pain.

Gareth

In my experience, whenever infertility is discussed, there are two basic assumptions made, over and over. The first is that it's the woman's problem; that the infertility is most likely hers. The second is that a couple have left it too late to try to conceive (again, the issues here are centred around the woman). When we were going through it all, people went straight to my wife to ask her how she was, and find out what was happening. I can't recall anyone approaching me to see if I was OK. Certainly, I was never asked if our issues were down to me – the male factor.

When you tell people that around 50% of conception difficulties are caused by male factor infertility, they're shocked. In the UK about 35% of men are sub-fertile, and 2% of men suffer with azoospermia (me included), which is the absence of sperm in semen. This can be due to an obstruction, total absence, or a number lower than 500,000 sperm per 1ml of semen.[2] Male infertility is called andrology. It's a big deal. But the word itself, and the world of male factor infertility it covers, is a well-kept secret.

Before my diagnosis, I never stopped to consider male infertility – that the root cause of our issues might be me. Nor had I known another man who'd faced that diagnosis. I was a part of the blind spot.

A major reason for this must be that men don't generally talk about such personal, difficult things in their lives. They never have and they still find it difficult today. If something isn't talked about, or heard, then it's the assumptions that are out there, not the facts, or the feelings.

From a man's perspective, it seems that our fertility issues are very tightly linked to those of masculinity. I can 100% say that as soon as I was diagnosed, I felt less of a man, like my primary function for being here had been taken away.

I was extremely lucky to have a supportive wife, but no amount of reassurance from her was going to change how I felt about myself. In true male style, I hid my head in the sand and avoided the whole thing. We existed like this for several months. Neither of us could talk about it, not fully. I fell back on what I knew worked. Support for my wife. Losing myself in my work. Anything to avoid what was really going on, the pain I was increasingly feeling. Eventually we fought about it, cleared the air and made a plan. If only I had managed to be more open from the start… But it doesn't work like this, not with the way things are around infertility today.

Men I talk to now share numerous reasons for finding it difficult to talk about infertility and what it makes them feel. One of the main ones is that we feel it's the man's job to be there as support for their partner; be their tower of strength. To achieve this we suppress our own feelings, because showing feelings is to show vulnerability, or weakness. Exactly, we think, what our partners don't need.

Then there is the embarrassment, or the shame part. It took me a full nine years after my diagnosis to get anywhere close to accepting it, to get over the instinctive shame of infertility, so that I could talk freely about it. I just couldn't face the personal facts, and the risks of breaking down in the face of all those questions from other people.

It seems so naturally different for women. They find it much easier to open up to each other, gain the support they need.

When I was checking some internet sites during our treatment, I was overwhelmed that 99% of contributors were female. My voice, it seemed, was lost – even when I was ready to talk. Online forum talk, amongst women, was about very specific women's issues – drugs, protocols, clinics, etc. – and shared feelings around those issues. There was no opening for me amongst all this. And if I did join in, then my contribution might lead to misinterpretation, or upset, from my wife.

For me, Facebook was the answer. Already it was a presence in my life, and I decided to use it to reach out to other men. With my wife's support, I started a closed group on Facebook, for men.[3] The ease of security settings meant I could create a space where members were verified, and once joined up, their names and posts hidden to the outside world. I knew this was key to getting men to join, that without this sense of privacy and security, they would continue to find it difficult to talk.

The page gives them all a platform to post, talk, vent their frustrations, seek and offer advice – all amongst their fellow men who know and understood what they are going through.

Initially I founded the group for me. I badly needed the conversation and support. But increasingly I became driven by the idea of help. My hope was if I could help one other man, the site was worth it.

To my surprise, men began to discover the page and gradually more and more people joined. As the membership grew, so did the diversity and experience of our conversations. It's been fantastic to see posts from men who only a few weeks previously were reluctant to share their problems and feelings, even with their closest friends or family.

Its unique pull is undoubtedly its men-only membership, and in today's world of equality, that has met with some opposition, from women who want to join. But it just couldn't function as it does if it were a mixed gender site. Its maleness is exactly why it works, and the more members and posts we get, the happier others are to contribute.

Acceptance of male infertility is growing. Slowly, more and more men are finding that it's OK to talk, and increasingly, there are professional support mechanisms being put in place. Fertility Network UK[4] have campaigned to assist men where needed, and dedicated andrology clinics are opening up. This is all positive progress. But we still have a long way to go, before men feel that they can naturally open-up and seek the support they need.

John

After failing to get pregnant, my wife and I both decided to do some tests through the NHS. I've never been ill in my life, so when I went into my local surgery to pick up the results, I didn't expect a problem. A doctor I didn't know told me he was very doubtful I would ever be able to father a child. The test paper had some minus numbers and a zero and a one, and it all looked a bit bleak. He wasn't the best communicator and failed to explain anything clearly. I left the surgery feeling pretty decimated and thought it was game over.

A few weeks later, we both went back and saw another doctor. He put a very different spin on it and said there was always a chance that something could be done, with the help of assisted pregnancy. And he told me what my problem was – a total lack of sperm mobility, although the sperm count was actually average.

It was then that we embarked on the whole assisted pregnancy route. After initially starting to do all this through the NHS, I was advised to go privately by a friend. It was quite a financial outlay but there was something about the NHS waiting and procedure that hadn't filled me with hope. Money was not a question, at least not in our minds, and I was quite happy to spend as much on the mortgage as it was going to take. We were lucky to have this financial choice.

Assisted pregnancy became the centre of everything in our lives. We tried to get through infertility as a couple and my wife always referred to it as our problem, not just mine. But I felt quite a bit of shame around it, and didn't really want anyone to know about it.

We were recommended to see Dr Taranissi, at his private clinic ARGC, and Zita West, a fertility expert. Looking back, both were good decisions. I felt I was in good hands.

First they needed to work out exactly what my problem was. Early on in the process, Zita West introduced me to a fantastic doctor called Sheryl Homer (who became known as the sperm expert!). It took quite a bit of investigative work before she found out exactly what was wrong, unique in its own way. She discovered I have a varicose seal in my left testis, which means that as soon as sperm arrives, it dies off. Most likely, Sheryl thinks, the blood circulation is blocked and so the temperature and/or chemical environment is wrong for sperm to thrive. But there was some hope: a few of the sperm she saw under the microscope were moving just a little, although at this stage, we didn't know whether they were fertile or not.

I then had some DNA tests, a prostate examination and many other tests. There was nothing wrong apart from the mobility issue.

I was now presented with a choice. Either I could have an operation to remove the varicose seal, in the hope that my sperm would return to normal. Or we could try ICSI[5], where in a cycle of IVF, a lively looking sperm could be injected into one of my wife's eggs. But since my sperm were so immobile, there wasn't much confidence around this route. I was all up for the operation as I felt it was like getting the car fixed. I met the surgeon and he filled me with confidence. However, Sheryl (the sperm expert) – a fantastic person throughout our story – rang me up to warn me off the operation, since she was concerned about other problems it might cause. She said she had an idea she'd like to try, although it was a long shot. She suggested a series of ejaculation tests to see if my sperm's movement increased if it was fresher. There might be fewer of them after several ejaculations, but there was a chance they might move more.

Masturbation on demand became a regular part of all this. Three times, one after the other, proved quite difficult. I needed a lot of imagination...

A few weeks later, during my wife's first cycle of IVF, I remember looking down the microscope – after a third ejaculation – and seeing that one of my sperm was moving around. So they used it to fertilise one of my wife's eggs. And to our amazement and delight, within a day or so it started to divide. So I was fertile, and now we were in with a chance. Sheryl told me she knew of another man whose case was very similar to mine. His sperm turned out to be infertile, so I felt incredibly lucky. My wife's pregnancy went well and we had a baby girl. It was our first IVF attempt, which was pretty amazing.

About a year later, we decided to go again, and now we started to experience the miserable side of infertility treatment. Our second IVF attempt failed to make my wife pregnant, and the third attempt resulted in a very painful ectopic pregnancy, ending with an operation. After all this she was emotionally very fragile. The hormone-induced changes really affected her and she was in tears much of the time, in quite a desperate state.

Throughout all the treatment, she found the self-injecting very tough, particularly the pregnancy hormone injections you have in the first, vulnerable stages of early pregnancy, to try and keep it going. The injections were painful and left big bruises. All this for someone who had a fear of needles.

I had to keep working during this whole period, and when I wasn't there, she didn't really have any support. Her family was uninvolved and friends were always busy. And I can now see, looking back, that my wanting to be secretive about it was a block to the support that she needed. We lacked a third person, to confide in and trust.

Infertility and its effects can really damage a relationship. We already had one child, so imagine going through all this without that one bit of luck. I'm not sure if we would have survived as a couple.

Now into her mid 30s, it felt like it was harder to get pregnant. Our fourth attempt seemed like it was OK, although the pregnancy blood test 'numbers' had fluctuated a little which wasn't a good sign. My wife was given a different kind of hormone injection, a stronger one, and the bruises from these injections lasted for ages.

But we went for our three-month scan and we were told all was good and the foetus was as it should be. We were so thrilled and again, felt incredibly fortunate.

But it wasn't to be. Unfortunately, my wife had a very late miscarriage. We were devastated. The pain was terrible and the whole thing was incredibly upsetting. To this day, I still feel like I didn't handle the emergency situation very well. I remember feeling scared at the hospital – we were staying up in Preston, and had to deal with everything away from home.

Afterwards, my wife's confidence was shattered. That was our last IVF attempt. Thankfully, she went for some counselling, but it took a while for her to regain some emotional and physical balance.

I still feel guilty about what she had to go through for something that was essentially my problem. But we feel incredibly lucky to have our daughter.

Leigh

The infertility journey can be a lonely one, whether as a couple or in those moments when you feel like you're so alone. Actually, you're far from alone, although being told this is of little comfort when you're in the thick of it. It wasn't to me, when my wife (R) and I started to have tests after two years of zero natural conception. We sought help, were diagnosed with unexplained infertility, and after four failed cycles of IUI (Intrauterine Insemination), faced IVF as our next step. At that time, I was very much in a place of Why me? Why us? It felt like we'd been singled out, made to struggle with something as basic and natural as creating our own family. The world became a more difficult and bitter place.

It began to drive an emotional wedge between my wife and I. Also between us and our closest friends who were starting to have children. Yes, we were thrilled for them, but they were difficult to be around too. My work performance suffered. As did my personal hygiene; self-respect; everything. I just didn't care.

Then came a tipping point when things all changed.

At work, I'm always in and out of customers' homes, and small talk is part of the job – finding the common ground between us to help fill in the gaps. And of course the usual kind of personal questions followed on, amongst them 'You got kids yourself?' Always hard this one, and sometimes their response to my flat-batted answer was the most painful thing to hear – 'Oh good, nothing but trouble' or 'Keep it that way, they'll ruin your life!'

Mostly I let these remarks go, ignored them for what they were. But one day I flipped – letting a customer know exactly what I thought of his comment and why I didn't have kids. Of course, they weren't to know, and the outburst led to an awkward apology and explanation.

I came home and spoke to R about my day, angered by people's insensitive and thoughtless comments. We knew it wasn't intentional. More a general lack of awareness, their simply not knowing how painful childlessness can be. But, we thought, maybe our silence was a part of the problem. Perhaps we could help? We decided to speak out.

At first this was to our family and close friends, in person. We put people in the picture, and talking about it helped hugely. Then to our wider circle of friends, through the magic of Facebook.

We found two Facebook groups to get involved with. One for both myself and R, a local support group for people attending the same clinic that we were. The other was a just-for-men infertility group – men from all over the world. Sharing experiences, advice and feelings with a whole mix of different guys, all of them one way or another in the same boat as me, has been incredibly valuable. Both supportive and cathartic, at different times.

Eventually we started our own blog, both of us – hugely helpful to us, and hopefully to others as well.

Around this time, I started to channel some of my frustrations into running – in turn, leading to help a charity[4]. I felt healthier in body and mind, found a fresh outlook on things. Answers to those previously difficult conversations at work became, 'Actually we're going through IVF at the moment.' No more hurtful follow-up comments. And the best thing – sometimes people were genuinely interested in what we were going through. We were getting back in our control, and it became an easier life to lead.

There is no clinical diagnosis that can totally fix unexplained infertility. But I was doing more to fix what I could. I knew from initial tests that I had low motility and morphology. And I knew that getting active would help this. I added rowing and basketball to the running. I gave up alcohol and started to take Wellman pre-conception tablets. It seemed to do the trick.

So that was me sorted. Or so I thought…

But what I hadn't reckoned on was being made to feel so *invisible* – once we were up and going with IVF. It still angers me now, and so much of it could have been avoided.

It wasn't R that was making me feel invisible, far from it. It was the process, the clinic, the language used, the manner of some of the staff. Of course, it made sense to label R as the patient – nearly everything that was happening in an IVF cycle was happening to her. But after years of going with R to appointments, and the staff knowing us well, I thought I'd be more included; that we'd be treated more as a couple. But at every scan, consultation, test – it was always R that was addressed, her name that was called out. I was demoted to follower, barely spoken to at all.

The obvious exception was when it was time for me to get a sample together. Then, for a brief role (a key one!), I was addressed directly.

Of course, many of the staff were absolutely lovely. But at these crucial times, when we needed to be strong, as a couple – and craved to be treated as such, particularly by the professionals – the general trend, particularly on the administrative side, was to focus only on R, and to sideline me.

And going unseen didn't stop at the hospital. Many times friends (even family) would ask, 'How is R doing? Must be so awful for her.' Thanks for asking, I'd think back, it's not great for me either. Yes, every woman involved in IVF gets the rawest deal! And I know it's not meant; that it's cultural, not personal. But the norm around fertility treatment, just like it so often is around pregnancy, is to over-focus on the woman; to lose sight of the other half, and therefore of the couple at the heart of the matter.

As a gender, we men are not the best at sharing, at letting our guard down. But we need every bit of help we can get. Only a slight shift in our direction, especially from healthcare professionals to lead the way, would make such a difference, not just to us, but to couples – both partners, in it together, for each other.

Actually, that invisibility (and inequality) I felt helped push me into taking action and getting back some of that control I mentioned earlier. I took the lead on our Facebook & Twitter sharing, did some vlogs, got involved with Fertility Network UK and signed up to as many media requests as I could.

But all that public side of things was secondary to what really mattered – my support for R. Helping to regain control also meant, we decided, that I would co-manage her drugs and the administering of her injections. It was probably the most intimate thing that we could share during our cycles, and I'm glad I had the chance to experience it.

Today, lots of male-aimed campaigns, from testicular cancer to mental health, suggest talking to a professional, should you feel the need. I did, and it's something I would do again. In the coming years, when things have calmed down, R and I have talked about starting a support group in our area. It's badly needed. So many people are coming up against these kinds of issues.

As I write this, I'm happy to say that our second round of IVF was successful. We're expecting a baby in a few months' time. Hard for some to read, I know, caught in the heartache-wreckage of yet another unsuccessful cycle. I don't mean it to be. I just want to put the idea out there that sharing your experiences – speaking out and cutting through the invisible, in whichever way you feel is best – really does help to limit the damage.

Philip

A colleague has just walked over and shown me his 20-week scan pictures. Of course I say I'm delighted for him. I can now, because I have two girls, thriving and very much alive. I'm getting used to having those convivial, jokey conversations about pregnancy and childbirth. All the scan pictures tend to look the same: the dotted outline of the spine; the patches of dark that the sonographers are able to identify with practised ease – 'there are the four chambers of the heart' – although they could be anything. (The similarity – you're not supposed to say this, but you do think it – to the xenomorph in *Alien* is striking, particularly when the poor thing suddenly twitches.)

The three pictures he shows me on the flimsy paper take me back to those empty years of IVF. I dreaded our own scans, when we were hoping in vain for a heartbeat after eight weeks. Seeing an empty sac, the pause of the sonographer or our gynaecologist, followed by that well-practised line, 'I'm sorry, it's not good news.' Then finally, obsessively scanning every day of our pregnancy, until our children were safely delivered. Sweaty palms, adrenaline and dread. 'Have you had a 4D scan? It's so realistic,' people would ask. Listen, we thought. We just never want to do another scan, ever again.

I don't have particular insights or advice on infertility. All I know is that the eight years it took for us to have children were like climbing a series of mountains. We would crest a rise expecting the summit but see yet another peak, suddenly finding ourselves right back at its base. Waking up at 4am, with a dizzying sense of falling, thinking everyone else is having children; we're being left behind. Today I am over those mountains (or whatever metaphor works better), and I would like to be able to forget it all. But of course I can't.

For eight years we were members of unofficial clubs – the Expecting Club, the Suddenly Not Expecting Club, the Miscarriage Club, the Stillbirth Club – with all the membership perks…Feeling like the ghost at the banquet when gathered with friends and their new children, the effort in maintaining those happy, fixed grins. The lurch of resentment, or a brief and shameful stab of a baser emotion, quickly suppressed, when friends announced new pregnancies. Turning off films mid-way through because the subject matter turned to pregnancy, or infertility (we needed an extra rating: don't view if you are trying desperately to have children).

For escapism, we watched some piece of trash called *Hellboy II*. The lead character, a grotesque red-skinned demon, ended up pregnant with a lovely pair of twins. Immediate end of film. It was all-consuming.

Some vignettes from those eight years:

Attending the Stillbirth and Neonatal Death Support meetings – as intense as they sound. We gathered in North London in the living room of its local coordinator (bizarrely he collected airline seats and we sat in those). We had lost our son G at 32 weeks, a stillbirth. For the months afterwards it felt as though someone had turned the colour down in the outside world. I struggled on with work and wished a colleague would stop using the term stillborn project to refer to an office issue.

A 25 litre sharps bin, purple and yellow – it sat in the corner of what was our shrine to lost hopes – the nursery; back then, a room firmly in quote marks. It was full of junk, full of unhappiness and at one point an unpacked buggy that one day had to be quietly spirited away. The bin filling up with blood-thinning heparin shots, mini plastic all-in-one syringes. An accompanying pile of empty packets of Thyroxine, Metformin, Hydroxychloroquine, Prednisolone steroids – taken to counter the body's immune reaction, or so the theory goes. We built up quite the search history on Google: what does bleeding three weeks post implantation mean? Chances of pregnancy after ectopic? The way those searches effortlessly auto-completed gave me a sense we were far from alone.

Endless meetings with gynaecologists, those plumbers of the medical world – unblocking fallopian tubes, flushing them with coloured fluid to check their viability. Feeling the world narrow to a few seconds as the consultant waved the sonogram wand around (usually an internal wand for those early scans). I am a diehard atheist but I even remember hedging my bets in one scan and vaguely offering a pact to the Supreme Being if *He* could arrange a heartbeat (he didn't, that time).

In 2014 we had twin girls. Our numbers came up, or something equivalent in the medical world, and suddenly that part of the journey was over. I'm a Dad now, so I can relegate those years spent trying to a corner of my mind and focus on getting on with life. But the slightest thing can take me back, and of course I can't forget G. We were parents long before we were… Parents.

I read a book by Elizabeth McCracken, 'An Exact Replica of a Figment of My Imagination'[6], that helped us through those months after our stillbirth. She summed it up perfectly for me in her last lines: 'I am happy but something is missing. I am happy and something is missing…'

12
Afterword

If I'd known, back then, all that I know now about fertility treatment, and our limited chances of success, especially around endometriosis, would I have embraced it with such open arms? Might we have got to adoption as our eventual route forward any faster? Daft speculation, obviously. And most probably, I guess we'd go down the same time line of treatment events if we were starting over. But that's all I sometimes question, broadly speaking, around IVF. I don't question the ethics of fertility science and the direction it's going in, or that current sense of priority it has over adoption, any more now than I did then. Yes, there are some better fertility doctors out there than others, wherever we go for our treatments. But in the several years since our first attempt, I have never challenged what I thought back then, that the progressive role of science in helping people overcome their infertility is largely a force for good.

It's good – although difficult when you're in the thick of it – to get a wider perspective on where this extraordinary new-life science is going, what it could offer infertility sufferers of the near future. Today, however one may feel about its ethics, reproductive science is making significant strides forward. Here's just a few examples of breakthrough fertility science from recent years that made the news.

The first has far reaching implications for couples undergoing IVF treatment. Genetic modification of embryos, commonly referred to as genetic editing these days, has just had a big shot in the arm. Dr Kathy Niakan, researching at the new Francis Crick Institute in Kings Cross, London, won approval from the HFEA[1] to undertake some editing of donated embryos (January 2016). Not surprisingly, China got there first, but had limited success in its attempts to mend a faulty embryo gene (2015). From Dr Niakan herself: 'We would really like to understand the genes needed for a human embryo to develop successfully in a healthy baby. The reason why it is so important is because miscarriages and infertility are extremely common, but they're not very well understood.' She aims to analyse a fertilised egg's first few days of development, from one cell to around 250 cells. As per ethical practice, and law, her batches of eggs will be destroyed after use (we're still years away from being able to implant genetically edited eggs back into a womb). Of course, her work will have its vociferous critics, those that see research like this as the latest steps towards the legalisation of GM babies. Last word to Sir Paul Nurse, Crick Director, outlining the implications of this momentous advance to everyone failing to conceive, or achieve a full, live term: 'Understanding how a healthy human embryo develops will enhance our understanding of IVF success rates, by looking at the very earliest stages of human development, one to seven days.'

The second is not new exactly, but recent developments are. A new kind of cell screening on pre-transfer five-day-old embryos, to see if they had the correct genetic set (23 chromosomes from the mother and 23 from the father) was found to significantly improve IVF success rates. Twenty weeks after transfer, 42% of the women screened using the current methods were pregnant, compared with 69% of women with the new screening. Overall, pregnancy success rate was improved by up to 65%. Nick Haan, leading the project at the Cambridge-based biotech company BlueGnome, summed up his team's work: 'For the first time, 24-chromosome screening and single-embryo transfer has the potential to become the default standard of care for all IVF cycles worldwide.'[2] I can see this on the IVF menu in the not-too-distant future, a significant development on chromosomal screening already practised today. How exciting, when it becomes real. Just one fertilised egg returned. The one out of the batch that stands a much better chance of maturing.

And the third, to do with the brave new world of stem cell research, will also draw as much controversy as it does excitement. Researchers have discovered that it is possible to find the stem cells in women's ovaries that go on to produce eggs – and will quite easily do so under lab conditions.[3] The clever bit was in isolating exactly the right stem cells that were destined for egg production, by finding a protein that was only present on the surface of these cells. Not yet, but one day in the future, it might be possible therefore, to make an unlimited supply of a woman's eggs, for the benefit of her own fertility treatment, and perhaps for that of her donor supply, too. And if that happens, then one of the founding theories of fertility – that a woman is born with all the eggs she will ever produce – could be turned upside down. There are cells in her ovaries that really are capable of creating more eggs. Astonishing! Of course, this kind of science, the stuff that uses *our* eggs, is strictly beyond the ethical pale. So, here's where we reach into the cage of laboratory mice…The cells were found to grow when they had been packed in human ovarian tissue and grafted inside mice. And when the tests were replicated using just mice – their stem cells and sperm – fertilisation was successful, and so too was the growth of embryos. Professor Allan Pacey[4], a fertility expert at the University of Sheffield, told the BBC that the study 'shows quite convincingly that women's ovaries contain stem cells that can divide and make eggs…Not only does this re-write the rule book, it opens up a number of exciting possibilities for preserving the fertility of women undergoing treatment for cancer, or just maybe for women who are suffering infertility by extracting these cells and making her new eggs in the lab.'

Exciting stuff, and all this before we get into the whole area of artificial wombs or the stem cell making of sperm. All these are big, biomedical science events that will have huge meaning, not just for men and women with health and fertility issues, but for our wider society. Imagine for a moment: stem cell eggs and sperm created in a lab; gestation in a glass womb[5]; no pregnancy (although naturally occurring feelings of being pregnant will be induced with hormonal drugs, as will breast milk); no birth trauma…All of it watched over by a doting mum and dad beginning to re-define their gender and parenting roles on a playing field levelled out as never before. Who the hell goes back to work first in that scenario! (Just for the record, science is perfectly capable of allowing men to breast feed too, should they want to. After all, we have milk ducts, just as women do, and mammary tissue and nipples, plus oxytocin and prolactin, the hormones responsible for milk production…)

But where do we stand? How do such visions of fertility science make us feel? As the red tops would shout, What price a baby? One thing is certain. The stage is awkwardly set, over the coming years of fast-forward science, for a long-lasting battle. The march of science – drummed on as much by the drug companies as our unquenchable thirst for human progress – versus the outrage of those whose religious sensibilities around the sanctity of life's beginnings feel so affronted. It's in the US, amongst the growth of the religious/ political right, that the battle cries will be loudest. Soon after he came to office, President Obama lifted the ban on the use of discarded embryos collected during IVF cycles being used for stem cell research. A lot of Republicans and folks of various religious persuasions will want to slap that ban straight back on, now that Trump is at the wheel. The lines in the sand are clearly drawn (like they are over abortion). On the one side is science, and a person's right to choose, and on the other, simply put, is God (the God side accusing the other of playing that very same God). And although both sides have a very different viewpoint on where human life starts, they both, ironically, begin with *life* at the very centre of their vision.

Personally, I find the advance of fertility science just as gripping to read and think about as the advances in the treatment of cancer or Alzheimer's or any other illness. I recently did some filming with a science researcher working in the field of neurology. I asked her about the presence of science progress in our lives. It wasn't the obvious answer, the one about combatting diseases, or steering us towards cleaner, planet-saving technology. Countries that promoted and prized science research, she said, gave us all the priceless opportunity of becoming questioners, not believers. Which in turn means we're likely to make better, more informed decisions. What a reassuringly weighty thought that is. As a couple, we chose the helping hand of science to try and fix our problem, treatment that was available to us, in our time. It's still pretty much the same today, several years later, give or take some fine-tuning. But ten, twenty, fifty years into the future, science will have its chances to move us on, as a force for good. That's if we allow it to, and if we can exercise enough care over its progress, and to whom it is available.

In the end, it will still come down to choice. Most likely, if it's available and approved, and if we can get our heads around it, then we'll be able to choose it. And this seems right. Would we choose to deny any other kind of sufferer – a diabetic, or someone with dementia for example – a tried and tested development in treatment? I don't think so. And infertility, with all the suffering that it can bring, is certainly a condition demanding a similar kind of respect. So, let careful and qualified science stick to its guns. It's good to have it there, if we want it.

One keynote on the development of infertility treatment: cost. In July 2013, news broke that IVF could, potentially, become cheaper.[6] Conventionally, IVF labs control the all-important acidity levels of embryos with expensive carbon dioxide incubators, medical grade gas and purified air. A lab in Belgium has tested a much cheaper approach, coming up with a kitchen cupboard mix of citric acid and bicarbonate of soda to produce an acceptable CO_2 environment. The lab claims that first-round tests produced a pregnancy rate of 30%, about the same as standard IVF. And that if these techniques are combined with the use of cheaper egg stimulation drugs, the costs of IVF could be substantially cut – by up to 80% in some cases. More affordable versions of IVF will have a huge impact worldwide. Not just in the West, amongst us, but in areas of the developing world where infertility is a big issue – socially and economically – and where IVF treatment has virtually no presence.

Attitudes are, slowly but surely, changing around infertility. As we learn more about its minefield of likely causes – environmental chemicals and pollutants, sexually transmitted diseases, detrimental diet and lifestyle, stress and delayed choice around pregnancy – and as we come to see it more as the illness it is (at last, it is classed as such[7]), so there'll be a wider acknowledgement and understanding of what it means. We need infertility to be a bigger deal, for it to be more visible, particularly as it sits as closely as it does to one of our hottest global potatoes – population.

Certainly, there are many more clinics open for business today, ready to meet the growing global demand, with their offers and results far more visibly sold. If you opened the same Family Values newspaper supplement as I did the other day you can't fail to have noticed a whole raft of clinics soft-selling their wares, in amongst all the other pop-family-topics of the day (education, sugar and salt, things to do outside and screens and teens, etc.). There was one half-page spread from a UK clinic[8] offering fertility day retreats and fertility yoga. Another full pager by Spanish clinic Dexeus[9], famous for producing the first in vitro baby in Spain some 30 years ago, then for two world firsts in the 1980s: first frozen embryo pregnancy and first donor egg baby. Finally, a half-page splash for a top clinic[10] in the Czech Republic. In one supplement! (Two of these, and hundreds of other overseas clinics showcased elsewhere, reflect the growing trend of people – increasingly motivated by lower costs and in some cases less stringent regulations – who are seeking their treatments outside of the UK.[11])

The whole world of infertility is more on the map, more in the everyday language. There's even an annual UK (in)Fertility Show held at London's Olympia, now in its eighth year and visited by 3,500 people.[12] (The Baby Show in October; The Fertility Show and Sexpo UK in November. Olympia has got it well covered!)

The likelihood is we'll make braver strides in the world of adoption, too. There'll be more campaigning for it, more initiatives to shift some of the underlying preconceptions and fears that surround it. Already, the UK has begun to look much more closely at adoption guidelines pioneered and accepted as the norm in the US – more openness and more flexibility around ethnicity and placement. I don't think we will let science and its fertility treatment outmanoeuvre adoption as the go-to infertility solution any more than it already does now. We have too many children in care needing permanent homes to let that happen. Texas is a big place, but last year they adopted a third more children than in the entire British Isles. That can't be right. We need a bigger, braver process.

Some of the breakthroughs described here, science or social, weren't on the main road map when I started this account. Nor were the number of support and counselling help routes that are around today. This is all bright news for people going through it, now and in years to come. Because whether infertility is on the rise or not (and this is much debated), it's a problem for which people are increasingly seeking more help.

Today, that's over three million couples in the UK alone, somewhere in excess of 50 million worldwide – a whole lot of people who thought they would have their baby when they were good and ready, exactly as per their script.

Endnotes

INTRODUCTION

1. Taken from www.hfea.gov.uk. The Human Fertilisation and Embryology Authority is the UK statutory and regulatory body in the Assisted Reproduction sector, answering to the Department of Health. See also Chapter 3, THE HELPING HAND OF SCIENC, note 7, for a fuller account of HFEA remit and role. Figures are taken from the HFEA's 'Fertility Treatment 2014-2016 Trends and figures' report (the latest UK fertility treatment figures available at the time of writing). www.hfea.gov.uk/media/2544/hfea-fertility-treatment-2014-2016-trends-and-figures.pdf. Also see HFEA's 'State of the fertility sector: 2016-17'.

1 DOING WHAT COMES NATURALLY

1. Surprisingly (you might think), the causes of approximately half of infertility cases are traced to male infertility. A man's fertility, broadly speaking, relies on the quantity and quality of his sperm. Low sperm quantity, or low quality, will likely lead to a male reproductive problem. It is thought that 1 in 20 men's fertility is impacted by a low sperm number (although only one in every 100 men has an absence of sperm altogether). Most often, there are no obvious signs or symptoms associated with male infertility issues: ejaculated semen appears normal to the eye. Hence the need for medical tests. There are many thorough accounts of male infertility causes – most often they are to do with production or transport of sperm – and what can be done to overcome the problems. For example www.andrologyaustralia.org.

One of the experts on Andrology (the medical science that deals with male health, particularly relating to the problems of the male reproductive system and urological problems unique to men) in the UK is Professor Allan Pacey BSc, PhD. It is now broadly accepted (but still little known and talked about) that whilst a man of forty or over may be very capable of fathering a child, his sperm might also be of less value to his partner and his child (in terms of its DNA), than when he was thirty or twenty years of age. Simply put, men are likely to become less effectively fertile the older they get. Dr Pacey has written much about the decreasing sperm quality in men over forty years of age, and the increased likelihood of problems with their children's health if conceived later in their lives (Down's Syndrome, for example, schizophrenia or autism spectrum disorders). 'There have been conflicting theories to explain why the children of older fathers are at increased risk of some medical conditions… So scientists have focused on the question of whether testicles become less efficient as men age, allowing errors or mutations to creep into the sperm genome. This is the first study to firmly establish that random mutations across the genome rise significantly as men age. That this may be possible should not be a surprise: sperm are produced quite quickly (about 1,000 with each heartbeat) and by the age of 50 the sperm precursor cells in testicles will have divided more than 700 times, with the potential for error each time…'

2. The Natural Fertility Clinic operated at Hospital of St. John and St Elizabeth, 60 Grove End Road, St. John's Wood, London NW8 9NH.

See also THE HELPING HAND OF SCIENCE for further notes on 'natural fertility' & 'soft' fertility treatments.

3. The IAC (Intercountry Adoption Centre), since 1997, has been the only specialist provider of overseas adoption services to prospective adopters. More recently (still called IAC but more widely known as the Adoption Centre) it has become a full-service adoption agency to people considering both domestic and intercountry adoption. Its mission statement: 'IAC's mission is to place children from all parts of the world, both in the UK and overseas, in loving families and to work in a fair, transparent and professional manner with all individuals who seek our professional services.' www.icacentre.org.uk.

4. The Hague Convention on Protection of Children and Co-operation in Respect of Intercountry Adoption (referred to as The Hague Adoption Convention, or in adoption circles, the Hague Convention). This is an international convention focusing on the human rights of children, with regards to adoption, child laundering, and child trafficking. It came into force on 1 May 1995. Concerning international adoption, the main objectives of the Convention are: to establish safeguards to ensure that intercountry adoptions take place in the best interests of the child and with respect for his or her fundamental rights as recognized in international law; to establish a system of co-operation amongst Contracting States to ensure that those safeguards are respected and thereby prevent the abduction, the sale of, or traffic in children; to secure the recognition in Contracting States of adoptions made in accordance with the Convention. As of March 2013, the Convention has been ratified by 90 countries, UK and USA included. 'Intercountry adoptions shall be made in the best interests of the child and with respect for his or her fundamental rights… Each State should take, as a matter of priority, appropriate measures to enable the child to remain in the care of his or her family of origin.' Inevitably, The

Hague Adoption Convention is having the effect of slowing down numbers of intercountry adoptions.

2 BEAR TRAPS

1. www.endometriosis-uk.org is a helpful UK site for all things endometriosis.
2. The London Women's Clinic is a state-of-the-art IVF and Fertility treatment centre. www.londonwomensclinic.com.

3 THE HELPING HAND OF SCIENCE

1. Assisted Reproduction & Gynaecology Centre (ARGC). www.argc.co.uk.
2. Much has been written about Dr Taranissi, a leading UK fertility expert. This Telegraph article offers a relatively balanced introduction. www.telegraph.co.uk/health/healthnews/9383167/Mohammed-Taranissi-interview-we-help-nature-to-achieve-what-its-meant-to-achieve.html.
3. Create Health offer 'a natural and safe approach to fertility'. www.createhealth.org. Dr Geeta Nargund is Founder and Medical Director. She is also lead consultant in reproductive medicine, St George's Hospital NHS Trust, London.
4. 'Soft IVF' aims to minimise the effects of IVF on a woman's health, reducing the risk of ovarian hyper-stimulation syndrome. Unlike conventional IVF, she can be fit and ready enough to try again, on her very next cycle. Weaker doses of drugs are used, and the cost per cycle reduces accordingly, sometimes by less than half the rates charged for more typical IVF. Although success rates are not as high as in conventional IVF (between 10 and 20% less, depending on age range), it's an appealing and gentle approach which is gaining support as a viable option, both for younger women with time on their side, and for older women wary of the effects of strong drugs on the quality of their dwindling egg supply. There's a good introductory article about soft IVF at www.telegraph.co.uk/health/women_shealth/7726034/A-softly-softly-approach-to-IVF-offers-women-fresh-hope.html.
5. Dr Nargund has strong views on conventional IVF, views that are gaining ground in an NHS always looking to economise. As said, she is an inspiring fertility doctor – pragmatic as much as she is principled and bold. A fertility expert whose primary concern is for the medical, social and economic wellbeing of the women being treated (a recent campaign of hers is to get fertility/infertility learning embedded into secondary school sex and relationship teaching). 'I am not in the business of proscribing life choices to anyone. The myriad circumstances of individuals and families who seek to

start a family make nonsense of the idea that one size (or age) will ever fit all. What I absolutely do stand for is the power of education and knowledge. With accurate data on fertility, women can make informed choices at every stage of their life and career. Women do not wish to be fobbed off with lies and half-truths. The only way they can make educated choices is to be educated.'
www.theguardian.com/society/2015/jun/03/choices-facing-women-who-want-children.

6. New Labour made significant progress within the realms of NHS infertility treatment. The aim for up to three cycles of IVF to be freely available to all women deemed with a reasonable chance of success was introduced (current guidelines suggest this means women between the ages of 23 and 39), and still holds good today, as the goal (despite inequality in its availability in some parts of the country). It was a groundbreaking acknowledgment of the very serious issue infertility is, the suffering it can cause, and the help that medical science can readily provide, if sufficiently supported. As referred to in 5, above, the NHS is finding it tough to offer one round of IVF, let alone three. In November 2015, the Independent ran an article titled 'RIP IVF?' NHS cuts to fertility treatment, it explained, could deny thousands of possible parenthood. www.independent.co.uk/life-style/health-and-families/health-news/rip-ivf-nhs-cuts-to-fertility-treatment-will-deny-thousands-parenthood-a6717326.html. It reported Mid and North East Essex have become the first Clinical Commissioning Groups in the UK to stop funding IVF (except in exceptional circumstances). Other Groups are considering following them. The article reports that figures published 2nd Nov 2015 by campaigning group Fertility Fairness show that just one in five CCGs provide three cycles – a drop of 6 per cent since 2013 – with fewer than one in four offering two cycles. The number of CCGs offering only one cycle has risen to 57 per cent – exacerbating the postcode lottery in fertility treatment as more couples are priced out of parenthood. The worry is that with private IVF treatment averaging around £5,000 per cycle, many people will be forced out of the IVF loop.

7. HFEA, Human Fertilisation Embryology Authority. Since 1991, the HFEA has licensed and regulated all IVF treatment and research in the UK. Its role is to represent, inform and protect us, patients and all, in the arena of fertility practice and research. The HFEA offers a rational, best practice view on what's going on, with regular updates as to its position on IVF treatment and research developments – medical, ethical and regulatory. The more contentious and sensitive issues that inevitably crop up in the IVF world are well covered in these statements (regarding the news on the number of UK IVF pregnancy

terminations, for example, 7th June 2010) and can be a positive counter read to some of the other, more alarmist media coverage. The HFEA makes available a free booklet supporting people on the fertility treatment journey. And its site runs a series of patient stories, a few of them written by courageous women whose IVF years have not given them the child they so wanted. The HFEA's role is also to support the infertility clinic business, particularly in the light of so many women seeking infertility services overseas (donor eggs in Italy, or Spain, for example, where women are paid more for donating eggs, so there's more of them). In recent years, the government has considered plans to disband the HFEA and split its regulatory duties across another commission and authority (part of plans to cut NHS administrative costs by over a third). As yet, not carried through. The HFEA has not always had a smooth relationship with the private clinic sector, particularly ARGC. But as a reliable bank of facts and perspectives, established over twenty years of public trust, it will be a hard act to follow.

8. Follicle-stimulation hormones, FSH. Controls the reproductive processes of the body. A rise in FHS levels triggers ovulation.

9. www.zitawest.com.

10. For example www.ncbi.nlm.nih.gov/pmc/articles/PMC3962314/ and www.nhs.uk/news/2007/January08/Pages/AcupunctureandsuccessofIVF.aspx.

4 DRUMMING UP SUPPORT

1. facebook.com/groups/mensfertilitysupport. This is a terrific men-only support group, started by Gareth Down, who found himself suffocating around the lack of opportunity to talk to other men about the infertility he and his partner were going through. Gareth has done much media work to promote awareness and support around male factor infertility. See Chapter 11, OTHER VOICES, Gareth, for his story behind this site.

2. The Independent, 8th July 2006.

3. For example, the idea that we're placing a growing and over reliant faith in IVF as a medical solution for infertility, or as a reason to wait, voiced by fertility expert Dr Gedis Grudzinskas. 'IVF: The Uncomfortable Truth.' www.theguardian.com/lifeandstyle/2010/jul/03/ivf-fertility-infertility-gedis-grudzinskas.

4. 'The New Couple: The Ten New Laws of Love' by Maurice Taylor, Seana McGee. Published by Thorsons Element. ISBN 13: 9780007195329.

5. 'Writing my way through cancer' by Myra Schneider. Jessica Kingsley

Publishers. ISBN 1-84310-113-0.

6. Churchill was known to finish many a wartime phone call with KBO. 'Keep buggering on' in longhand.

5 THEY'RE IN THE FREEZER!

1. See full details in latest HFEA report 'Fertility Treatment 2014-2016 Trends and figures'. The key findings in this report are as follows:

- Between 1992 and 2016, there have been over 1,100,000 IVF treatment cycles in UK licensed clinics.
- In 2016, there were just over 68,000 IVF treatment cycles, resulting in 20,028 births. This was a 4% increase from 2015 to 2016.
- Since 2014, frozen IVF treatment cycles have increased by 39%.
- In 2015, birth rates for frozen cycles exceeded fresh for the first time.
- In 2016, 31% of IVF treatment cycles were frozen, up from 27% in 2015.
- 12% of IVF treatment cycles used donor eggs, sperm or both.
- The birth rate per embryo transferred (PET) was 21% for all cycles.
- The birth rate PET for frozen cycles was higher than for fresh cycles for the second year in a row (22% frozen, 21% fresh).
- 41% of IVF treatment cycles were funded by the NHS.
- 42% of IVF patients were under 35, with 58% over 35.

2. Post transfer blood tests look for progesterone and Beta HCG levels. Beta HCG is the pregnancy hormone produced by the cells of the tiny embryo as it starts to implant.

3. See same HFEA 2014-2016 fertility treatment report referenced above. Includes guide to treatments offered by UK clinics, including PGS, preimplantation genetic screening, where cell(s) are removed from an IVF embryo to test for chromosomal normality/abnormality.

4. http://haveababy.com. Sher Fertility/SIRM is one of America's largest and most successful fertility clinics. A good source of current US thought leadership in the fertility treatment field.

5. Dr Geoffrey Sher, Executive Medical Director and co-founder of SIRM, is an internationally renowned expert in the field of assisted reproductive technology (ART).

6. www.zitawest.com/ivf/reproductive-immunology.

7. haveababy.com/infertility-information/endometriosis

8. 'Some fertility clinics offer tests and treatments which are based on the idea that immune cells in your body can reject a foetus, preventing a successful pregnancy. This is an area of medicine called reproductive immunology and

the treatments are called immunosuppressive therapies. The theory behind reproductive immunology has been widely discredited, and there is no evidence that immunosuppressive therapies improve your chance of getting pregnant.' There is a full explanation of the HFEA's position at this site. The 'widely discredited' stance taken by the HFEA is questioned by many, indication of the controversy referred to surrounding reproductive immunology.

6 VEGAS, THE FINAL THROW OF THE DICE

1. Since our trip to Vegas for treatment, the idea of 'medical tourism', even 'IVF holiday' has gained more than a foothold. And not just in Vegas. Clinics across Europe, including Eastern European countries, as well as in Asia, America, South Africa and the Middle East offer infertility sufferers a full range of attractively packaged treatments. See also Chapter 12, AFTERWORD, note 10.

8 WHEN ENOUGH IS ENOUGH

1. Since 2011, there has been a successful push by the HFEA in the UK for law change around egg donation. Financial reward has been introduced for women donors. From www.hfea.gov.uk. 'Egg donor payment: as an egg donor you can receive compensation of up to £750 per cycle of donation, to reasonably cover any financial losses incurred in connection with the donation, with the provision to claim an excess to cover higher expenses (such as for travel, accommodation or childcare). This in turn aims to slow the rising trend of egg tourism to other donator countries, where the process is more straightforward and accessible.'

2. There's a balanced overview of surrogacy on the HFEA site https://www.hfea.gov.uk/treatments/explore-all-treatments/surrogacy/.
There are several helpful surrogacy hubs in the UK, for both would-be parents and surrogates, for example www.surrogacyuk.org (this one run by both sets of stakeholders and recognised by the Department of Health and the British Medical Association). An article at www.bbc.co.uk/news/magazine-28864973 covers some of the alarm-bell aspects of surrogacy, as well as one or two success stories. 'In the UK you cannot pay for a woman to have your baby, regulation is loose and arrangements depend entirely on trust. Demand for surrogates far outstrips supply.' Published at the same time as BBC R4 programme 'The Report, Surrogacy' (21st August 2014), it begins in the UK, then swoops in on India, where many British Asians head, fuelling an international surrogacy business worth $1bn in India alone.

3. Latest HFEA figures clearly show the rising trend of in vitro cycles involving

a donor egg. See full details in latest HFEA report 'Fertility Treatment 2014-2016 Trends and figures'.

9 ADOPTION, THE LONG WAY HOME

1. Latest 2017 figures can be seen at corambaaf.org.uk.
(Coram BAAF Adoption & Fostering Academy.)
And a full breakdown of all children in care, adoption and fostering 2017 statistics at www.gov.uk/government/statistics/children-looked-after-in-england-including-adoption-2016-to-2017.
2. Form F3. An assessment form filled in by prospective adopters. This is completed, stage by stage, during the course of the home study, under the guidance of the assigned social worker.
3. 'Adoption without Fear' by James L. Gritter, M S W. Gazelle Book Services Ltd (Dec 1989). ISBN-10: 0931722713 ISBN-13: 978-0931722714.

10 THE AFTERWARDS OF INFERTILITY

1. Resolve, the National Infertility Association, is a helpful resource in understanding more about secondary infertility (SI). Defined by Resolve as 'The inability to become pregnant, or to carry a pregnancy to term, following the birth of one or more biological children. The birth of the first child does not involve any assisted reproductive technologies or fertility medications.'
https://resolve.org/infertility-101/medical-conditions/secondary-infertility/.
2. An article worth reading on SI.
http://www.telegraph.co.uk/women/womens-health/5088578/Secondary-infertility-One-is-not-enough.html.

11 OTHER VOICES

1. www.fertilityfriends.co.uk.
2. www.malefertility.co.uk.
3. facebook.com/groups/mensfertilitysupport/.
Mentioned before in Chapter 4, DRUMMING UP SUPPORT, but worth another one here.
4. Fertility Network UK. www.infertilitynetworkuk.com. 'Advice, support, understanding.'
5. ICSI. There's a clear explanation on the HFEA site: 'Intra-cytoplasmic sperm injection (ICSI) differs from conventional in vitro fertilisation (IVF) in that the embryologist selects a single sperm to be injected directly into an egg, instead

of fertilisation taking place in a dish where many sperm are placed near an egg.'

6. 'An Exact Replica of a Figment of My Imagination' by Elizabeth McCracken. Jonathan Cape; ISBN-10: 022408710X ISBN-13: 978-0224087100.

12 AFTERWORD

1. The news of HFEA's approving of Dr Kathy Niakan's research was published widely across relevant publisher sites, in early Feb 2106. For example www.nature.com/news/uk-scientists-gain-licence-to-edit-genes-in-human-embryos-1.19270.

2. Published in Molecular Cytogenetics, 2nd May 2012.

3. BBC 26th February 2012. www.bbc.co.uk/news/health-17152413.

4. Professor Alan Pacey BSc, PhD, Department of Human Metabolism, Academic Unit of Reproductive and Developmental Medicine, Sheffield University (see Chapter 1, DOING WHAT COMES NATURALLY, note 2).

5. The process described here is called Ectogenesis – the development of embryos in artificial conditions outside the womb.

6. For example www.bbc.co.uk/news/health-23223752.

Stuart Lavery, Director of IVF at Hammersmith Hospital, said the study had the potential to have a big impact globally. 'This isn't just about low cost IVF in west London, this is all about how you can bring IVF to countries which have unsophisticated medical services where infertility has an incredibly low profile. They've shown that using a very cheap, very simple technique that you can culture embryos and you can do IVF. The weakness of the study is they've done it in a big lab in Belgium, so they need go out and do the same study in Africa now. But if this is real potentially you're talking about bringing IVF to corners of the world where there is no IVF. This is enormous, the potential implications for this could be quite amazing.' Note: this IVF treatment did not provide for specialist processes like sperm injection into eggs (ICSI) or extensive chromosome screening.

7. In 2010, The World Health Organization (WHO) and the International Committee for Monitoring Assisted Reproductive Technologies (ART) released a new international glossary of ART terminology. For the first time, infertility itself is classed as a recognised illness: 'A disease of the reproductive system defined by the failure to achieve a clinical pregnancy after 12 months or more of regular unprotected sexual intercourse.'

8. Awakening Fertility. www.Awakeningfertility.com (including 'Natural Fertility' programmes).

9. Dexeus. en.dexeus.com. (Open for business, even in Spanish August!)

10. Reprofit. www.reprofit.eu.

11. Worldwide, between 20,000-25,000 couples seek fertility treatments outside of their home countries. See breakdown of who's travelling where and for what treatments at

https://en.wikipedia.org/wiki/Fertility_tourism.

A dip in the online waters results in a huge amount of editorial and commercial material to read on the subject, from journalists, clinics and patients themselves. Again, the information within 'Considering fertility treatment abroad' at www.hfea.gov.uk is worth reading. Since cost is such a big influencer in the decision-making process, it's now openly written about, in the same tone as any other major household outlay. For example, this one about cost, at www. money.co.uk/guides/fertility-treatment-abroad-can-you-save-money.htm.

12. www.fertilityshow.co.uk. 2017 saw the ninth year of this show. There were 60 seminars from some of the world's leading fertility specialists, and over 100 exhibitors (UK and overseas) with doctors, clinicians, practitioners and fertility experts on their stands. Open to all, 'whether you're just thinking about starting a family or have been trying for ages...' So well attended is this November event, an ongoing sister event is now held in Manchester, in March www.fertilityshow.co.uk/manchester.

About the Author

A quest for shared understanding and greater clarity around fertility is at the root of this book, as is his own personal experience of the subject.

Having always written poetry (his work has been nominated in the National Poetry Competition), this is his first book.

Born and raised in rural Worcestershire, he now lives in London with his wife and young son. He co-runs his own film production company.

Printed in Great Britain
by Amazon